Absolutely Paleo!

The 150+ Recipe Paleo Blueprint

Table of Contents

Cave-Italy Flatbread

Dinner Recipes

Cave Beef Sliders
Simple Zucchini Rollatini
Spicy Chicken Bite Supreme
Bacon Quesadilla
Easy Gyro and Avocado Tzatziki
Cave Meatball Sub
Easy Sausage and Peppers
Primal Chicken Souvlaki and Paleo Tzatziki
Paleo Cheese Steak "Sandwich"
Crisp Spinach Salad Delight
Ultimate Kelp Noodle Stir-Fry
Shrimp Taco Supreme
Healthy Paleo Veggie Burger
Spicy Mango Fried "Rice"
Chicken "Noodle" Soup
Gazpacho and Paleo Tortilla Chips
Easy Paleo Chili
Seared Tuna Salad
Jamaican Cave Jerk Patty
Primal Chicken Pot Pie
Cave BBQ Pork Sandwich
Smoked Salmon Eggs Benedict
Half Shell Oysters
Almond Crusted Pan Seared Scallops
Primal Style Marinated Baby Octopus
Primal Shrimp Stuffed Squid Delight
Oysters and Pancetta Gratin

Sage Sausage Dinner Buns
Paleo New Yorkshire Puddings
Tropical Guava Refresher Salad

Pastries Recipes

Almond Pizza Crust
Pizza Naan
Paleo Pizza Pita
Soft Baked Pretzel
Caveman German Chocolate Cake
Quick Paleo Coconut Ginger Crisps
Paleo Pecan Blast Shortbread Cookies
Cinnamon Raisin Cookies
Cocoa Cafe Biscotti
Choco Pecan Chess Pies
Paleo Chocolate Mandarin Scones
Cashew Crew Belgian Waffles
Ultimate Apple Upside Down Cakes
Primal Flourless Chocolate Cake
Apple Dump Supreme Muffins
Easy Pumpkin Spice Cakes
Quick Paleo Biscuits
Classic Gingerbread
Curry Spice Bread
Banana Nut Bread Delight
Simple Squash Muffins
Cave Kefir Rolls
Classic Everything Bagels
Cave-Cocoa Gingerbread
Decedent Apple Bread

Honey Nut Sweet Buns
Blueberry Blast Scones
Pumpkin Muffins
Easy Cinnamon Raisin Bread
Paleo Cinnamon Raisin Bagels
Paleo Chocolate Bacon Donut
Easy Raw Coconut Cookies

Raw Recipes

Simple Homemade Almond Milk
Simple Homemade Coconut Milk
Simple Homemade Flaked Coconut Milk
Green Smoothie
Nature-Blast Smoothie
Paleo Spiced Pear Smoothie
Paleo Lemon Crush Refresher
Lime Cooler Crush Supreme
Cocoa Chutney
Maroon Ants-On-A-Log
Date Butter with Apples
Lemon Spotted Spring Salad
Pecan Blast Spinach Salad
Raw Blueberry Bars
Raw Paleo Creamy Fudge
Banana Cream Pie Supreme
Raw Goodness Ginger Cookies
Cashew Cream Chocolate Mousse
Zucchini Salad and Primal Tomato Sauce
Hot Tuna Tartare
Cashew Cream Avocado Hummus

Quick Raw Green Slaw
Nature's Tomato Soup
Smoked Salmon and Green Snacks
Kelp Noodle Salad and Cashew Sauce

Craving Recipes

Sweet Cinnamon Pretzel
Choco Banana Bites
Fruit 'N Nut Bars
Paleo Cocoa Cream Bun Delight
Honey Nut Bun
Chocolate Fried Pie Supreme
Green Cake
Lemon Treat Coconut Cake
Strawberry Blondies
Paleo Sugar Cookies
Primal Chocolate Cherry Brownies
Mixed Berry Trifle Delight
Carrot Cake Cookies
Chocolate Mousse
Paleo Plain Vanilla Pudding
Baked Donut
Paleo Avocado Banana Bread
Paleo Peach Cobbler
Primal Berry Treat Tart
Strawberry Sweet Cake
Orange Shortbread Cookies
Paleo Walnut Blast Cookies
Chocolate Mint Cookies

Primal Pistachio Pinwheel Cookies
Paleo Angel Cake Delight
Carrot Cake Cookie Bars
Lemon Spotted Muffins
Paleo Coconut Macaroons
Paleo Coconut Cake

Everyday Recipes

Cave Style Breakfast Buns
Green Club Muffin
Primal Corn Muffins
Paleo English Muffins
Coconut and Banana Pancake Supreme
Ultimate Bacon & Fruit Scramble
Paleolithic Egg Bread
Green Crush Smoothie
Red Berry Blast Smoothie
Strawberry Banana Swirl Shake
Cashew Butter Banana Sandwich
Strawberry Swirl Sandwich
Primal Beef Bun
Mighty Onion Crumpets
Jalapeño Lime Comfort Pretzel
Cave Style Thai Curry
Simple Cashew Curry
Easy Pesto Caprese Salad
Ultimate Primal Pad Thai
Zesty Clam Dish
Southwestern Chili
Paleo Broccoli Creamy Soup

Primal Raspberry Fusion Salad
Cave People Guacamole
Rugged Coconut Shrimp
Toasty Almond Cream Cakes
Classic Pineapple Upside Down Cake
Banana Bread Pudding Delight
Simply Sweet Potato Blondie Refresher
Coconut Cream Comfort Pie
Paleo Strawberry Bread
Primal Apple Cider Bread
Mandarin Pumpkin Coconut Bread
Garlic Goodness Rolls
Savory Tomato Rolls
Blueberry Blast Blondies

Why Choose the Paleo Lifestyle?

If you haven't been living under a rock, you've probably already heard of the Paleo Diet. Celebrities like Megan Fox are strong advocates for the Paleo lifestyle to keep fit and look great. But what exactly does eating Paleo mean?

The Paleolithic Diet, or Paleo for short, is a nutritional approach that tries to mimic our ancestor's way of eating. It's much more of a lifestyle than a diet. The primary goal of eating Paleo is not necessarily weight loss, so the word "diet" may not ring properly to those who are already fit and seeking to improve their performance in sports or simply to be healthier. However, it is believed that most people would highly benefit from adopting a Paleo lifestyle.

Several millennia ago, our caveman ancestors ate whatever they could hunt or gather: fruit, meat, seeds, nuts and vegetables. This has been the basis of human nutrition throughout evolution. That is, until 10,000 years ago when humans discovered agriculture. This led to a more sedentary lifestyle, and foods such as grains, legumes and dairy became a major part of our diet. They are easy to grow and harvest, they quickly curb hunger and provide tons of energy.

However, 10,000 years is merely the blink of an eye on the evolution timeline, which spans several million years. It is now thought that this short period since the agricultural revolution has not been long enough for our bodies to adapt to all these new foods. This phenomenon has grown in importance in the last half-century, as processed foods and junk became deeply rooted in the Standard American Diet. Soda, burgers, pizza and fries are making matters much worse and destroying the bodies of millions of people every day.

Since our bodies cannot process the products of agriculture (dairy, grains and legumes) the same way they process berries, nuts and seeds, the partially undigested foods create many health problems such as obesity, cancer and chronic pain. These foods also contain toxins that cause chronic inflammation levels throughout the body. Eating Paleo means returning to a more ancestral way of eating. It eliminates the worst offenders (processed foods) along with dairy, legumes and all grains.

Before you start wondering how long it will take you to starve to death without these foods, have a look at Paleo recipe books. You'll find plenty of delicious ideas to make meat, veggies, eggs and nuts the focus of your meals. You'll even find tons of recipes for amazingly decadent Paleo desserts. Nut flours, coconut flour and seeds allow you to make bread substitutes. You can replace pasta with zucchini noodles. You can make "cheese" with soaked nuts. By now, you should have a pretty clear idea of what the Paleo lifestyle is all about.

Fresh or dried fruits, vegetables, nuts, eggs, seeds, meat and coconut oil are all Paleo staples. The guidelines for the Paleo diet are based on what we think the ancient hunter-gatherers would have been eating. Making the Paleo switch will have you exploring new ways to prepare your favorite foods. Going Paleo will give you more energy along with reducing your risk of modern diseases such as obesity, cancer, inflammation and dementia. Better yet, you will find it much easier to lose stubborn fat! While it is by no means a low-fat nor a low-carb diet, the foods consumed on the Paleo diet will transform your body for the better. There is no need to count calories, fat grams or carbs. There is no weird preparation involved, and there are no unnatural ingredients either.

You will finally enjoy food in its natural, wholesome way, just like nature intended it. You will also find that making time to cook isn't actually that hard. You might even (gasp!) discover a newfound love for cooking. For many people, taking on the challenge of cooking Paleo is actually enjoyable. You will be taken through an unmatched culinary journey as you reinvent your favorite classics or tweak new recipes to make them Paleo. This book will be your guide as you get started with Paleo cooking. It contains a ton of delicious Paleo-approved recipes that you can serve to your family with zero guilt. Finally, a diet that allows you to have bacon and not feel bad about it!

Foods to Avoid

You will want to avoid:

- All grains: these are not part of the Paleo lifestyle. Cavemen didn't have access to grains before agriculture and we are not designed to digest them properly without excessive stress on our digestive system. This includes rice, wheat, barley, rye, spelt, amaranth, corn, millet, quinoa, kamut, etc. Replace grain-based flours with coconut and nut flours for your baked goods. Not only will the protein, fiber and fat content increase, but the taste will be subtle and quite pleasant. Make sure you follow the guidelines for Paleo baking, as you cannot simply substitute a cup of whole wheat flour for a cup of almond flour.

- Legumes such as soy, edamame, lentils, chickpeas, beans (black, red, white, kidney, pinto, etc.), yellow and green peas. However, yellow and green string beans are fine.

- Dairy: milk, cheese, yogurt, butter, ice cream, etc. This is another extremely inflammatory group of foods that should be avoided. However, clarified butter (ghee) is generally accepted by the Paleo guidelines. This special butter has been stripped of everything but its milk fat contents, making it minimally inflammatory.

- Processed sugar and regular salt: avoid these at all costs. Nothing good ever comes from consuming these unnatural and dead foods. Opt for more natural options such as Celtic Sea salt or Himalayan pink salt, agave nectar, maple syrup, honey and stevia extract. These all fit the Paleo guidelines when used with moderation.

- High amounts of fruit: this can be detrimental to health because of their fructose content. Fructose is another inflammatory food. Most Paleo guides will agree that one or two pieces of fruit per day is acceptable, but try not to go overboard with it.

- Processed foods: if it comes in a box, a can or a package, it's probably not Paleo. Some exceptions apply, such as Paleo energy bars and some canned veggies that contain no added salt, sugar or preservatives. Frozen produce is fine, as long as it is not packaged with chunks of garlic butter or any other non-Paleo ingredient. Junk and fast-food fall into this category as well. Make your own food at home so you can control the quality and quantity of ingredients.

- Potatoes: these are pretty controversial. Some Paleo followers will eat them because they could theoretically have been dug up by a caveman half a million years ago. However, potatoes did not exist in their current form during the Paleolothic Era. Regular white potatoes contain some of the inflammatory toxins (lectins and saponins) that the Paleo diet tries to avoid. So, while they're certainly a fairly nutritious whole food, they are not recommended for those who go Paleo. Instead, load up on sweet potatoes, which are free of these toxins and generally accepted by Paleo followers. Be careful not to overdose on sweet potatoes if you need to lose weight, as their sugar and starch content is high.

Lunch Recipes

Chicken Dumpling Bun

Prep Time: 15 minutes

Cook Time: 20 minutes

Servings: 4

INGREDIENTS

Dumpling Bun

1 cup tapioca flour

1/4 - 1/3 cup coconut flour

1 cage-free egg

1/2 cup warm chicken stock

1/4 cup coconut oil

1/4 cup applesauce

1 teaspoon apple cider vinegar

1 teaspoon baking soda

1/2 teaspoon onion powder

1/ 4 teaspoon garlic powder

1/2 teaspoon Celtic sea salt

Filling

8 oz boneless chicken (breasts, thighs, etc.)

1 small carrot

1 small celery stalk

1/2 teaspoon dried thyme

1/4 teaspoon ground sage

1/2 teaspoon ground black pepper

1/2 teaspoon Celtic sea salt

INSTRUCTIONS

1. Preheat oven to 350 degrees F. Line sheet pan with parchment paper or coat with coconut oil. Heat medium skillet over medium heat and lightly coat with coconut oil.

2. Add chicken stock to small pot and heat over medium heat.

3. For *Filling*, dice carrot and celery, fillet chicken in half, and add to hot oiled skillet with salt and spices. Sauté until chicken is cooked through and browned and veggies are softened, about 5 - 8 minutes. Remove from heat and set aside. Shred or dice rested chicken and mix thoroughly with sautéed veggies.

4. For *Dumpling Bun*, sift together tapioca flour, coconut flour, baking soda, salt and spices in medium bowl.

5. Whisk egg, applesauce and vinegar in small bowl. Whisk in warm chicken stock and coconut oil.

6. Add egg mixture to flour mixture and mix until well combined. Add 1 tablespoon coconut flour or water at a time if needed to form soft and slightly sticky dough.

7. Divide dough into 4 portions and flatten into round disks. Dust your hand or rolling pin with extra tapioca flour to prevent sticking.

8. Scoop chicken *Filling* into center of each dough disk and pinch edges of dough together to create round, sealed ball.

9. Place filled buns sealed side down on sheet pan and pat down slightly.

10. Place in oven and bake 20 minutes, or until edges are golden brown and dough is cooked through.

11. Remove from oven and let cool about 5 minutes.

12. Serve warm.

Cave-Mexican Shrimp Gazpacho

Prep Time: 35 minutes

Servings: 2

INGREDIENTS

Shrimp

10 - 12 large shrimp

1 - 1 1/2 cups lemon juice (about 8 lemons)

1/2 jalapeño pepper

Gazpacho

2 cups tomato juice (about 4 large tomatoes)

2 plum tomatoes

1/2 red bell pepper

1/2 red onion

1/2 cucumber

Small bunch fresh cilantro

2 garlic cloves

2 tablespoons raw apple cider vinegar(optional)

2 tablespoons raw oil (coconut, walnut, almond, sesame, etc.) (optional)

1 teaspoon ground black pepper

1 teaspoon Celtic sea salt

INSTRUCTIONS

1. For *Shrimp*, Peel, devein and remove tails from shrimp. Mince jalapeño and juice lemons. Add to small bowl and mix. Shrimp

should be completely covered in lemon juice. Place in refrigerator for 30 minutes, or until shrimp are opaque.

2. For Gazpacho, juice large tomatoes in juicer. Or add to food processor or high-speed blender and process, then strain into medium mixing bowl.

3. Peel cucumber and seed. Seed plum tomatoes. Seed, stem and vein bell peppers. Peel onion and garlic. Dice veggies and onion, and mince garlic. Add to tomato juice.

4. Add salt, pepper, vinegar and oil (optional). Mix well, then place in refrigerator.

5. Chop cilantro and set aside.

6. Remove shrimp from refrigerator and drain lemon juice and jalapeños. Rinse if desired.

7. Mix shrimp into tomato mixture. Pour into serving bowls and top with chopped cilantro. Serve chilled.

Easy Carrot Soup

Prep Time: 10 minutes

Servings: 2

INGREDIENTS

3 large carrots

1/2 cup fresh young coconut meat (about 1/2 young coconut)

1/4 cup raw pine nuts (or raw cashews)

1/2 - 1 inch piece fresh ginger

2 sprigs fresh cilantro

1 tablespoon coconut aminos (or raw apple cider vinegar)

1/2 teaspoon fresh cracked black pepper

Water (or coconut milk)

INSTRUCTIONS

1. Remove cilantro leaves from stems and add to highs-speed blender. Juice ginger, or peel and finely grate. Add to blender with pine nuts, coconut, and coconut aminos.
2. Juice carrots, or add to food processor or high-speed blender and process until smooth, about 2 minutes. Add enough water or coconut milk to reach desired consistency.
3. Pour into serving bowls and top with fresh cracked black pepper. Serve immediately.

Primal-Cali Turkey Burger

Prep Time: 5 minutes

Cook Time: 15 minutes

Servings: 4

INGREDIENTS

Paleo Soft Burger Bun

16 - 20 oz ground turkey

4 - 6 slices nitrate free bacon

1 avocado

1 heirloom tomato

2 ribs romaine lettuce (or preferred lettuce)

1/2 cup alfalfa sprouts

Celtic sea salt, to taste

Ground black pepper, to taste

INSTRUCTIONS

1. Preheat oven to 350 degrees F. Line sheet pan with parchment paper, or lightly coat with coconut oil. Or lightly coat 6 mini round cake pans with coconut oil. Heat medium skillet over medium-high heat.
2. Prepare *Paleo Soft Burger Buns* and place in oven.
3. While bread bakes, cut bacon strips in half and place in hot pan. Cook about 5 minutes, until browned and crisp on both sides. Set bacon aside.

4. Form ground turkey into 4 patties and place in hot pan. Reduce heat to medium. Sprinkle with salt and pepper and sear 4 -5 minutes on each side.

5. Cut lettuce ribs in half. Cut tomato into 4 thick slices. Slice avocado in half, pit and slice flesh in peel.

6. Remove *Paleo Soft Burger Bun* from oven and let cool about 5 minutes.

7. Slice bun in half and place lettuce on bottom bun, followed by tomato slice. Add burger patty, then 2 - 3 bacon strip halves, and a pinch of alfalfa sprouts. Top with a few slices of avocado and top bun.

8. Serve immediately.

Cave BLT

Prep Time: 10 minutes*

Cook Time: 20 minutes

Servings: 2

INGREDIENTS

Paleo Sandwich Bread

8 slices nitrate-free bacon

1 large tomato

2 ribs romaine lettuce

1/2 cup arugula leaves

1/2 cup baby spinach

Honey Mustard

2 oz organic mustard

2 tablespoons sweetener*

INSTRUCTIONS

1. Preheat oven to 350 degrees F. Lightly coat 6 mini round cake pans with coconut oil. Or lightly coat loaf pan with coconut oil. Heat medium skillet over medium-high heat.

2. Prepare *Paleo Sandwich Bread* and place in oven.

3. While bread bakes, cut bacon strips in half and place in hot pan. Cook about 5 minutes, until browned and crisp on both sides. Remove skillet from heat and set bacon aside.

4. Shred romaine lettuce and toss with spinach and arugula. Thinly slice tomato. Mix mustard and sweetener in small mixing bowl.

5. Remove *Paleo Sandwich Bread* from oven and let cool about 5 minutes. Slice and spread with *Honey Mustard*.

6. Layer bottom bread slice with half lettuce mix, tomato slices and crisp bacon. Top sandwich with top bread slice and cut in half on the diagonal. Repeat with second sandwich.

7. Serve immediately.

*raw honey or agave nectar

Sweet Potato Fries and Ketchup

Prep Time: 5 minutes

Cook Time: 35 minutes

Servings: 2

INGREDIENTS

Sweet Potato Fries

1 large sweet potato

2 tablespoons coconut oil

1/2 teaspoon ground black pepper

1/2 teaspoon ground paprika

1/2 teaspoon Celtic sea salt

1/4 teaspoon cayenne pepper (optional)

Paleo Ketchup

4 oz (1/2 can) organic tomato sauce

6 oz (1 can) organic tomato paste

1 tablespoon apple cider vinegar

1/2 teaspoon garlic powder

1/2 teaspoon onion powder

1/2 teaspoon ground black pepper

INSTRUCTIONS

1. Preheat oven to 450 degrees F. Line sheet pan with parchment or coat lightly with coconut oil.

2. Peel sweet potato if preferred, but do not rinse. Slice sweet potato into 1/4 inch strips and add to medium mixing bowl with coconut

oil, black pepper, paprika and cayenne (optional). Toss potatoes until well coated.

3. Spread fries in well-spaced, single layer on sheet pan. Sprinkle salt over potatoes.

4. Place sheet pan in oven and bake for 10 minutes.

5. Carefully remove sheet pan and turn fries over with tongs or spatula. Place sheet pan bake into oven. Bake for another 10 minutes, or until golden and crispy.

6. While *Sweet Potato Fries* bake, add tomato sauce, tomato paste, vinegar, garlic powder, onion powder and black pepper to small pot.

7. Heat pot over medium heat and reduced for about 5 minutes, stirring occasionally.

8. Once reduced, remove pot from heat. Transfer ketchup to serving dish and refrigerate about 20 minutes.

9. Remove sheet pan from oven and serve *Sweet Potato Fries* hot with *Paleo Ketchup*.

Fish Sandwich and Easy Slaw

Prep Time: 20 minutes

Cook Time: 20 minutes

Servings: 1

INSTRUCTIONS

Paleo Soft Burger Bun

Crispy Fish

6 oz fillet white fish (cod, tilapia, catfish, etc.)

1/4 cup almond meal

1 egg

1/2 teaspoon ground black pepper

1/2 teaspoon Celtic sea salt

Quick Slaw

1/4 head cabbage (1 cup shredded)

1 small carrot

zest of 1/2 lemon

Juice of 1/2 lemon

2 tablespoons coconut oil

1 - 2 tablespoons apple cider vinegar

1 tablespoon sweetener* (optional)

1/4 teaspoon ground white pepper (or black pepper)

1 teaspoon Celtic sea salt

DIRECTIONS

1. Preheat oven to 350 degrees F. Line sheet pan with parchment paper, or lightly coat with coconut oil. Or lightly coat 6 mini round cake pans with coconut oil.

2. Prepare *Paleo Soft Burger Buns* and place in oven.

3. While bread bakes, heat small skillet over medium heat and coat with coconut oil.

4. For *Quick Slaw*, remove any tough outer leaves and core from cabbage. Shred cabbage and carrot. Add to medium mixing bowl with vinegar, coconut oil, sweetener, salt and pepper. Zest *then* juice lemon, and add. Toss to combine and place in refrigerator.

5. For *Crispy Fish*, beat egg with half of salt and pepper in small mixing bowl. Mix almond flour with remaining salt and pepper in small dish.

6. Coat fish fillet in egg then dredge in almond flour. Place fillet in hot oiled pan and cook about 3 minutes on each side, until crispy and golden but still juicy.

7. Remove fish from pan and drain on paper towels.

8. Remove *Paleo Soft Burger Bun* from oven and let cool about 5 minutes.

9. Slice bun in half and add *Crispy Fish*. Top with *Quick Slaw* and serve immediately.

*stevia, raw honey or agave nectar

Lamb Pot Pie Supreme

Prep Time: 15 minutes

Cook Time: 30 minutes

Servings: 4

INGREDIENTS

Filling

8 oz lamb

1 1/2 cup beef or vegetable broth

2 tablespoons tapioca flour

2 tablespoons coconut oil

2 chopped carrots

1 chopped celery stalk

1 bell pepper (yellow, orange or red)

1 small green tomato (or under ripe red tomato)

1 small onion

2 garlic cloves

1 inch piece ginger

1 tablespoon curry powder

1 tablespoon ground coriander

1 teaspoon ground cumin

1/2 teaspoon ground cinnamon

1/2 teaspoon black pepper

Pinch Celtic sea salt

Crust

1/3 cup almond flour

2 tablespoons coconut flour

3 tablespoons cold coconut oil (or cacao butter)

1 cage-free egg

3 - 4 teaspoons water

1/2 teaspoon turmeric

1/4 teaspoon Celtic sea salt

INSTRUCTIONS

1. Preheat oven to 400 degrees F. Heat medium pot over medium heat.
2. Add two tablespoon coconut oil to hot pot. Add lamb. Sauté about 5 minutes, then remove lamb with tongs.
3. Whisk in coconut flour until smooth. Gradually whisk in broth. Simmer about 5 minutes, whisking occasionally.
4. Peel and mince garlic and ginger. Chop carrots, celery, onion, bell pepper and tomato. Add to pot with salt, and spices.
5. Chop par-cooked lamb meat. Add lamb back to pot and simmer for 5 minutes. Remove from heat and set aside.
6. For *Crust*, add cold coconut oil to flours, turmeric and salt in small bowl. Cut fat into flour with fork until crumbly. Mix in egg and enough water to bring together tender dough.
7. Divide dough into 4 portions. Roll into balls and flatten into round disks large enough to fit over mini pie tins or ceramic ramekins with hand, then rolling pin.
8. Pour *Filling* into vessels and cover with crusts. Pinch edges of dough over edges of vessels to seal in liquid. Brush top of each pie

with coconut oil, coconut milk, or egg wash and sprinkle with salt. Use knife to cut a slit in the top of each pie.

9. Bake pot pies for about 15 minutes, until crust is golden.

10. Remove from oven and allow pies to cool for 10 minutes.

11. Serve warm. Or let cool completely and serve room temperature.

Ultimate Meatballs

Prep Time: 5 minutes

Cook Time: 20 minutes

Servings: 4

INGREDIENTS

16 oz (1 lb) ground meat (beef, pork, chicken, bison, or any combination)

1 cup almond flour

1 egg

1 garlic clove

1/2 small onion

1 teaspoon dried parsley

1 teaspoon dried oregano

1/2 teaspoon ground black pepper

1/2 teaspoon Celtic sea salt

Tomato Sauce

4 oz organic tomato sauce

4 oz organic crushed tomatoes

1 teaspoon dried oregano

1/2 teaspoon dried basil

1/2 teaspoon ground black pepper

DIRECTIONS

1. Preheat oven to 350 degrees. Line baking sheet with parchment or baking mat. Or prepare glass or ceramic casserole dish.

2. Pulse onion and garlic in food processor or blender until finely processed, but before paste forms. Or finely mince onion and garlic.

3. Beat egg in large bowl. Add ground meat, almond flour, spices and salt. Mix well with hands or large wooden spoon.

4. Form 18 - 24 meatballs with scoop or tablespoon, then roll in hands.

5. Arrange meatballs on lines sheet pan or in casserole dish and bake for 15 to 20 minutes, until golden brown and cooked through.

6. Add all *Tomato Sauce* ingredients to small pot and heat over medium heat. Stir and simmer about 10 minutes, until reduced and thickened.

7. Remove meatballs from oven. Toss with *Tomato Sauce* and serve hot.

8. Or allow meatballs and *Tomato Sauce* to cool, then pack in lidded containers. Serve room temperature.

Peach Pecan Primal Pie

Prep Time: 20 minutes

Cook Time: 20 minutes

Servings: 4

INSTRUCTIONS

Crust

2 cups almond flour

2 cage-free eggs

3 tablespoons coconut oil

1 tablespoon sweetener*

1/4 teaspoon baking soda

1 teaspoon ground cinnamon

1/2 teaspoon Celtic sea salt

Filling

2 peaches

1/4 cup dried apricots

1/4 cup pecans

2 tablespoons sweetener*

2 tablespoons water

1 tablespoon ground cinnamon

1 teaspoon vanilla

1/2 teaspoon ground ginger

DIRECTIONS

1. Preheat oven to 400 degrees. Line sheet pan with parchment or baking mat. Cover cutting board with parchment.

2. For *Crust*, sift almond flour into medium mixing bowl. Add baking soda, cinnamon and salt.

3. Whisk eggs and sweetener in small mixing bowl, then add to flour and combine. Slowly add coconut oil until malleable dough comes together.

4. Roll in plastic wrap or wrap tightly in parchment and refrigerate for 15 minutes.

5. Heat medium pan over medium heat.

6. Peel and pit peaches. Chop apricots, pecans and peaches. Add to hot pan with sweetener, spices and water. Sauté about 5 - 10 minutes, until peaches are tender and

7. Remove dough from refrigerator. Roll dough out on parchment covered cutting board to about 1/8 inch thick square with rolling pin. Use sharp knife or pizza cutter to cut dough into 4 squares.

8. Scoop equal portions of *Filling* into center of one side of each dough square. Fold bare half of dough over filled half. Press edges together, letting any trapped air escape. Crimp edges of dough together with fork. Repeat with remaining dough.

9. Arrange pies on lined sheet pan and bake 15 - 20 minutes, or until dough is golden and cooked through.

10. Serve immediately. Or allow to cool and store in air-tight container.

*stevia, raw honey or agave nectar

NOTE: Heat large skillet over medium heat , add 1/4 inch coconut oil, and fry pies 2 minutes on each side for traditional *Fried Pies*.

Sweet Potato Primal Pie

Prep Time: 20 minutes

Cook Time: 30 minutes

Servings: 4

INSTRUCTIONS

Crust

2 cups almond flour

2 cage-free eggs

3 tablespoons coconut oil

1 tablespoon sweetener*

1/4 teaspoon baking soda

1/2 teaspoon ground cinnamon

1/2 teaspoon Celtic sea salt

Filling

1 large sweet potato

1/2 cup dried dates

1/4 cup walnuts

1 cage-free egg

1 teaspoon vanilla

1 teaspoon ground cinnamon

1 teaspoon ground nutmeg

1/2 teaspoon ground black pepper

DIRECTIONS

1. Bring medium pot of lightly salted water to boil. Cover cutting board with parchment.

2. For *Crust*, sift almond flour into medium mixing bowl. Add baking soda, cinnamon and salt.

3. Whisk eggs and sweetener in small mixing bowl, then add to flour and combine. Slowly add coconut oil until malleable dough comes together.

4. Roll in plastic wrap or wrap tightly in parchment and refrigerate for 15 minutes.

5. Preheat oven to 400 degrees. Line sheet pan with parchment or baking mat.

6. Peel and dice sweet potato. Chop dates. Add sweet potato and dates to boiling water peaches. Cook about 10 minutes, until sweet potatoes are soft. Drain sweet potatoes and dates.

7. Add egg to medium mixing bowl. Add 1 tablespoon hot sweet potatoes to bowl. Mash briefly, then add second tablespoon. Gradually add all hot sweet potatoes and dates to egg. Mash and mix, careful not to scramble egg. Stir in vanilla, cinnamon, nutmeg and pepper.

8. Chop walnuts. Set aside.

9. Remove dough from refrigerator. Roll dough out on parchment covered cutting board to about 1/8 inch thick square with rolling pin. Use sharp knife or pizza cutter to cut dough into 4 squares.

10. Scoop equal portions of *Filling* into center of one side of each dough square. Fold bare half of dough over filled half. Press edges together, letting any trapped air escape. Crimp edges of dough together with fork. Repeat with remaining dough.

11. Arrange pies on lined sheet pan and bake 15 - 20 minutes, or until dough is golden and cooked through.

12. Serve immediately. Or allow to cool and store in air-tight container.

stevia, raw honey or agave nectar

NOTE: Heat large skillet over medium heat , add 1/4 inch coconut oil, and fry pies 2 minutes on each side for traditional *Fried Pies*.

Cave Blueberry Pies

Prep Time: 25 minutes

Cook Time: 20 minutes

Servings: 4

INSTRUCTIONS

Crust

2 cups almond flour

2 cage-free eggs

3 tablespoons coconut oil

1 tablespoon sweetener*

1/4 teaspoon baking soda

1/4 teaspoon ground cinnamon

1/4 teaspoon ground ginger

1/2 teaspoon Celtic sea salt

Filling

2 cups blueberries (fresh or frozen)

2 tablespoons sweetener*

1 teaspoon vanilla

1/2 teaspoon ground ginger

1/4 teaspoon ground black pepper

1/4 teaspoon Celtic sea salt

INSTRUCTIONS

1. Preheat oven to 400 degrees. Line sheet pan with parchment or baking mat. Cover cutting board with parchment.

2. For *Crust*, sift almond flour into medium mixing bowl. Add baking soda, cinnamon, ginger and salt.

3. Whisk eggs and sweetener in small mixing bowl, then add to flour and combine. Slowly add coconut oil until malleable dough comes together.

4. Roll in plastic wrap or wrap tightly in parchment and refrigerate for 15 minutes.

5. Heat medium pan over medium heat.

6. Add blueberries to hot pan with sweetener, vanilla, ginger, salt and pepper. Cook blueberries down for about 10 minutes, until juices thicken and reduce. Stir occasionally.

7. Remove dough from refrigerator. Roll dough out on parchment covered cutting board to about 1/8 inch thick square with rolling pin. Use sharp knife or pizza cutter to cut dough into 4 squares.

8. Scoop equal portions of *Filling* into center of one side of each dough square. Fold bare half of dough over filled half. Press edges together, letting any trapped air escape. Crimp edges of dough together with fork. Repeat with remaining dough.

9. Arrange pies on prepared sheet pan and bake 15 - 20 minutes, or until dough is golden and cooked through.

10. Remove from oven and serve immediately. Or allow to cool and serve room temperature.

*stevia, raw honey or agave nectar

NOTE: Heat large skillet over medium heat , add 1/4 inch coconut oil, and fry pies 2 minutes on each side for traditional ***Fried Pies***.

Banana Nut Blast Pies

Prep Time: 25 minutes

Cook Time: 20 minutes

Servings: 4

INSTRUCTIONS

Crust

2 cups almond flour

2 cage-free eggs

3 tablespoons coconut oil

1 tablespoon sweetener*

1/2 teaspoon baking soda

1/2 teaspoon baking powder

1 teaspoon ground cinnamon

1/2 teaspoon nutmeg

1/4 teaspoon Celtic sea salt

Filling

2 bananas

1/4 cup walnuts

1 teaspoon ground cinnamon

1/2 teaspoon ground nutmeg

1/2 teaspoon ground ginger

1/2 teaspoon ground black pepper

1 teaspoon vanilla

1 tablespoons sweetener * (optional)

INSTRUCTIONS

1. For *Crust*, sift almond flour into medium mixing bowl. Add baking soda and powder, cinnamon, nutmeg and salt.

2. Whisk eggs and sweetener in small mixing bowl, then add to flour mixture and combine. Slowly add coconut oil until malleable dough comes together.

3. Roll in plastic wrap or wrap tightly in parchment and refrigerate for 15 minutes.

4. Preheat oven to 400 degrees F. Line sheet pan with parchment or baking mat. Cover cutting board with parchment.

5. For *Filling*, peel bananas and finely chop. Finely chop walnuts. Add to medium mixing bowl with vanilla, spices and sweetener (optional).

6. Remove dough from refrigerator. Roll dough out on parchment covered cutting board to about 1/8 inch thick square with rolling pin. Use sharp knife or pizza cutter to cut dough into 4 squares.

7. Scoop equal portions of *Filling* into center of one side of each dough square. Fold bare half of dough over filled half. Press edges together and secure seal, letting any trapped air escape. Repeat with remaining dough.

8. Arrange pies on prepared sheet pan and bake 15 - 20 minutes, or until dough is golden and cooked through.

9. Remove from oven and serve immediately. Or allow to cool and serve room temperature.

*stevia, raw honey or agave nectar

NOTE: Heat large skillet over medium heat, add 1/4 inch coconut oil, and fry pies 2 minutes on each side for traditional *Fried Pies*.

Pumpkin Bacon Pancakes

Prep Time: 5 minutes

Cook Time: 15 minutes

Servings: 2

INGREDIENTS

1 3/4 cups almond flour

1 cup almond milk

1/2 cup pumpkin puree

2 eggs

1 teaspoon baking powder

2 teaspoons ground cinnamon

1 teaspoon vanilla

1/4 teaspoon Celtic sea salt

4 slices nitrate-free bacon

INSTRUCTIONS

1. Heat large skillet over high heat.
2. Chop bacon into 1/2 inch pieces. Add to hot skillet and brown. Stir occasionally with wooden spoon.
3. Whisk eggs in medium bowl. Then whisk in almond milk, pumpkin puree, vanilla and cinnamon.
4. Add almond flour, salt and baking powder. Whisk until smooth.
5. Once crisp, reduce pan to medium heat and remove bacon from pan, leaving drippings. Drain bacon bits on paper towel, then stir into pancake mixture.

6. Use ladle or dry measure cup to pour 1/4 cup of batter onto hot oiled skillet. Fit 2 or 3 pancakes comfortably, so they do not touch as they spread.

7. Cook until sides of pancakes are firm and batter bubbles up a bit. About 3 to 4 minutes.

8. Carefully flip pancakes with spatula and cook for additional minute, or until cooked through. Repeat with remaining batter. Pancakes will be slightly delicate, so flip and plate with care.

9. Serve warm. Top with topping of choice.

Easy Chicken Patties

Prep Time: 5 minutes

Cook Time: 10 minutes

Servings: 2

INGREDIENTS

8 oz chicken

1 cage-free egg

1/4 cup coconut flour

1/2 sweet onion

1 tablespoon apple cider vinegar

1 teaspoon ground black pepper

1 teaspoon Celtic sea salt

1 teaspoon paprika

1 teaspoon ground sage

1 teaspoon dried thyme

1 teaspoon fennel seed (optional)

1/2 teaspoon nutmeg (optional)

1 tablespoon water

Coconut oil (for cooking)

INSTRUCTIONS

1. Heat medium skillet over medium heat and lightly coat with coconut oil.

2. Grind chicken meat and peeled 1/2 onion to medium grind in food processor, bullet blender, or meat grinder. Or grind onion alone and add to pre-ground chicken in medium bowl.

3. Add apple cider vinegar, spices and 1 tablespoon coconut flour to ground chicken and onion. Mix well until combined. Form into 2 large or 4 small patties and place on plate.

4. Beat egg with water and pour egg wash over patties. Gently flip patties to get them evenly covered with egg wash. Take coconut flour and sprinkle over both sides of egg washed patties. Pat coconut flour gently into patties.

5. Place coated patties into hot oiled skillet and cook about 3 - 4 minutes, until golden brown and crisp. Flip and cook another 3 - 4 minutes, or until done.

6. Remove cooked patties from pan and drain on paper towel. Serve hot.

Turkey Bacon Club Salad Supreme

Prep Time: 10 minutes

Cook Time: 5 minutes

Servings: 1

INGREDIENTS

Salad:

4 slices turkey bacon

1 tablespoon coconut oil

1 heart of romaine lettuce

2 medium tomatoes, chopped

Dressing:

1 avocado

1/2 small white onion

1 small garlic clove

Juice of 1 lemon

Small bunch of parsley leaves

Pinch Celtic sea salt

Pinch ground black pepper

INSTRUCTIONS

1. Heat medium skillet to medium-high heat and add coconut oil.
2. Chop turkey bacon and add to skillet. Browned for 2 - 3 minutes on each side, until thoroughly cooked. Remove turkey bacon and preserve any leftover oil.

3. Rinse and dry heart of romaine, then chop. Dice tomato and toss with lettuce in large bowl.

4. For ***Dressing***, slice avocado in half, pit, and spoon flesh into food processor or bullet blender. Add peeled onion and garlic, lemon juice and parsley. Add excess coconut oil from pan. Process until smooth. Salt and pepper to taste.

5. Use tongs to transfer lettuce and tomatoes to plate. Sprinkle on turkey bacon, and drizzle with avocado ***Dressing***. Serve immediately.

Simple Paleo Cobb Salad

Prep Time: 10 minutes

Cook Time: 10 minutes

Servings: 1

INGREDIENTS

Salad:

2 slices natural ham

2 slices nitrate-free bacon

1 heart of romaine

1/2 cup watercress

1/2 cup spinach

1 medium tomato

1/2 avocado

1 cage-free egg

Dressing:

2 tablespoons coconut oil

1 tablespoon apple cider vinegar

1 tablespoon lime juice

1 teaspoon organic mustard (or powder)

1/2 avocado

1 small clove garlic,

Small bunch cilantro

Pinch Celtic sea salt

Pinch ground black pepper

Pinch paprika

Pinch cayenne pepper

INSTRUCTIONS

1. Bring small pot to boil with salted water. Heat medium skillet over medium-high heat.

2. Gently add whole egg to boiling water for about 7 minutes, or until hard boiled.

3. While egg cooks, chop bacon and ham. Add bacon pieces to skillet. Brown bacon for about 5 minutes, until crisp and cooked on both sides. Drain bacon on paper towel. Add ham to skillet just to warm, and remove skillet from heat. Stir to warm evenly.

4. Rinse and dry heart of romaine, spinach and watercress. Chop lettuce.

5. Dice tomato. Slice in half, pit and dice flesh of half of avocado. Reserve other half.

6. Drain warm ham on paper towel. Reserve leftover bacon grease.

7. Drain hardboiled egg and cool under running water for about 30 seconds. Peel egg and chop.

8. Peel onion and garlic. Then add all *Dressing* ingredients with reserved avocado half to food processor or bullet blender. Add reserved bacon grease (optional). Process until smooth. Salt, pepper, paprika and cayenne to taste.

9. Use tongs to plate lettuce mix. Drizzle salad with avocado *Dressing*. Add chopped tomato, eggs, bacon, ham and avocado in single adjacent lines across lettuce mix. Serve immediately.

Primal Crab Cakes

Prep Time: 5 minutes

Cook Time: 10 minutes

Servings: 2

INGREDIENTS

8 oz pre-cooked lump crabmeat

1 cage-free egg

1 lemon

1 teaspoon ground crab boil seasoning (Old Bay Seasoning™)

1 tablespoons fresh basil

1 tablespoon fresh parsley

1/4 cup almond meal

1 ripe avocado

Coconut oil (for cooking)

1. Heat large skillet over medium-high heat and coat with coconut oil.
2. Slice in half, pit and scoop flesh of half of avocado into medium mixing bowl. Preserve other half.
3. Chop basil and parsley and add to avocado. Zest lemon into bowl to taste. Cut lemon in 1/2 and squeeze about 1 tablespoon of juice into bowl, excluding seeds. Mash well.
4. Add egg to bowl blend. Add crabmeat, crab boil seasoning and almond meal. Mix gently but thoroughly.
5. Form 4 small or 2 large crabmeat patties, pressing firmly to help hold them together. They will be delicate.

6. Add crab patties to hot oiled for about 3 - 4 minutes. Carefully flip and continue cooking for another 3 - 4 minutes on each side, or until golden brown.

7. Drain crab cakes on paper towel. Slice reserved avocado. Plate crab cakes and top with sliced avocado. Drizzle with squeeze of lemon. Serve hot.

Acorn Squash 'N Eggs Delight

Prep Time: 5 minutes

Cook Time: 15 minutes

Servings: 2

INGREDIENTS

1 medium acorn squash

2 cage-free eggs

1/2 small sweet onion

Ground black pepper, to taste

Celtic sea salt, to taste

1 tablespoon apple cider vinegar

Pinch of cinnamon (optional)

Coconut oil (for cooking)

INSTRUCTIONS

1. Heat large skillet over medium heat and coat generously with coconut oil. Bring medium pot to simmer with salted water, plus apple cider vinegar.

2. Peel acorn squash and onion, and grate. Drain shreddings in paper towel, pressing out moisture.

3. Combine squash, onion, black pepper and salt in small bowl. Place 4 handfuls into hot well-oiled skillet. Spread lightly to create thin, crisp patties. Brown acorn hash patties for about 5 minutes, then carefully flip. Brown another few minutes until cooked through.

4. While squash finishes, gently crack 1 egg into simmering water. Let poach for about 1 minute, then scoop out with slotted spoon and carefully drain on paper towel, careful to keep yolk intact. Repeat with second egg.

5. Plate acorn patties, 2 per person. Sprinkle with cinnamon (optional). Top with lightly poached egg. Remove from heat and serve.

Beef Plantain Stir-Fry

Prep Time: 10 minutes

Cook Time: 15 minutes

Servings: 2

INGREDIENTS

8 oz grass-fed beef

1 sweet plantain

1 small yellow onion

1/2 red bell pepper

2 cloves garlic

1 Serrano pepper

1 teaspoon ground cumin

1 teaspoon chili powder

1 teaspoon paprika

Small bunch fresh cilantro

1/2 lime

Coconut oil (for cooking)

INSTRUCTIONS

1. Bring a medium pot to boil with lightly salted water. Leave enough room in pot for sweet plantain. Heat large skillet over high medium heat and coat with coconut oil.

2. To peel plantain, cut in half then careful make at least 4 slices through peel lengthwise. Get finger or butter knife under tough peel and pry off.

3. Cut peeled plantain cut into 1 inch pieces, then in half, forming half moons. Add to boiling water for about 5 - 8 minutes, or until tender but not mushy.

4. Stem and seed peppers. Peel onion and garlic. Dice beef into half inch cubes and add to medium bowl. Mince Serrano pepper and garlic, and add to beef. Sprinkle with cumin, chili powder and paprika. Mix with wooden spoon to avoid getting hot pepper oil on skin.

5. Slice onion and bell pepper and add to hot skillet. Sauté about 1 minute. Add seasoned beef to skillet. Sauté another 2 minutes to brown.

6. Remove plantains from boiling water and drain. Add to hot skillet and stir-fry all together for about 2 - 3 minutes, until beef is browned and cook to about medium-well and plantains are a bit caramelized.

7. Chop fresh cilantro. Remove skillet from heat and toss stir-fry with cilantro. Plate stir-fry and squeeze over lime juice. Serve hot.

Classic Tuna Spread

Prep Time: 5 minutes

Servings: 1

INGREDIENTS

7oz (1 can) chunk light tuna

1 avocado

1/2 small red Onion

1 carrot

1 celery stalk

1/2 Lemon

1/2 cucumber

Ground black pepper, to taste

Celtic sea salt, to taste

Paprika, to taste

INSTRUCTIONS

1. Drain tuna. Cut celery stalk in half, and preserve larger end. Peel onion. Slice avocado in half, pit and scoop out flesh into small bowl. Mash well.

2. Finely dice onion, smaller half of celery stalk, and carrot. Add to bowl, with spices to taste.

3. Add tuna to bowl, plus squeeze of lemon. Mix until combined and smooth.

4. Slice reserved half of celery stalk into sticks. Slice cucumber into 1/3 inch round.

5. Serve tuna in bowl with cucumber chips and celery sticks.

Classic Salmon Veggie Salad

Prep Time: 10 minutes

Cook Time: 10 minutes

Servings: 1

INGREDIENTS

Salad:

1 medium salmon fillet (or 2 oz smoked salmon, do not cook)

1 carrot

1/2 cucumber

8 asparagus stalks

1 cup cabbage

1/2 lemon

Dressing:

1 avocado

2 tablespoons coconut oil

1/2 lemon

1 small clove garlic

1 tablespoon fresh parsley

1 tablespoon fresh dill

Pinch Celtic sea salt

Pinch ground black pepper

Pinch paprika

INSTRUCTIONS

1. Bring small pot to boil with salted water. Heat small skillet over medium-high heat and lightly coat with coconut oil.

2. Parboil asparagus spears in boiling water for about 2 minutes. Then drain and shock in ice bath.

3. Lay salmon fillet skin-side down in hot oiled skillet. Cook about 3 minutes on each side. Season to taste, then squeeze lemon juice over fillet.

4. Shred or grate cabbage, carrot and cucumber. Drain cucumber in paper towel. Dry asparagus in paper towel and slice into 2 inch pieces. Toss veggies together.

5. Peel garlic and add all **Dressing** ingredients with squeeze of lemon and salt, pepper and paprika to taste to food processor or bullet blender. Process until smooth.

6. Plate shredded veggies. Remove salmon fillet and flake off meat over shredded veggies. Or lay smoked salmon slices over veggies.

7. Drizzle salad with avocado **Dressing**. Squeeze a little more lemon juice over salad. Serve immediately.

Mince Meat Pie

Prep Time: 20 minutes

Cook Time: 30 minutes

Servings: 8

INGREDIENTS

Crust

4 cups almond flour

2 cage-free eggs

1/4 cup coconut oil

1/2 teaspoon Celtic sea salt

Filling

12 oz grass-fed beef

2 sweet apples

2 tart apples

1 cup beef stock

1/4 cup sweetener*

Juice of 1 orange

Zest of 1 orange

1/4 cup arrowroot powder

1/4 cup apple cider vinegar

1 cup raisins

1/2 cup dried pitted dates

1/2 cup dried pitted prunes

1/2 cup dried cherries

2 teaspoons ground cinnamon

1 teaspoon ground nutmeg

1/2 teaspoon ground cloves

1/2 teaspoon ground black pepper

1/2 teaspoon salt

INSTRUCTIONS

1. Preheat oven to 350 degrees F. Heat large pot over medium-high heat and lightly coat with coconut oil. Lightly oil pie plate. Prepare 4 sheets of parchment.

2. Place beef in hot oiled pan and brown on each side for about 5 - 7 minutes, until just cooked through. Remove beef and set aside. Add beef stock to pot.

3. Mix all *Crust* ingredients together in medium bowl until dough forms. Divide dough in half and use rolling pin to roll dough between two parchment sheets into circles to fit about 1 inch over pie plate.

4. Press one dough circle into pie plate. Crimp edges to create small lip. Bake for 5 minutes, then remove and set aside.

5. Peel, core and grate or dice apples. Add to beef stock with sweetener, zest and juice of orange, vinegar, raisins, cherries, spices and salt. Dice beef, prunes and dates, and add to pot. Stir in arrowroot powder and thicken for a few minutes.

6. Once mixture comes together pour into par baked pie shell. Top with second dough sheet and crimp edges to fit into bottom crust.

7. Use sharp knife to slice top crust a few times for venting.

8. Bake pie for 30 minutes, or until crust is golden brown.

9. Remove from oven and allow to cool for about 20 minutes.

10. Slice and serve warm. Or allow to cool completely and serve room temperature.

*stevia, raw honey or agave nectar

Almond Butter Balls Delight

Prep Time: 10 minutes

Cook Time: 10 minutes

Servings: 12

INGREDIENTS

1/2 cup almond butter

1/2 cup almonds

1/4 cup cashews

1 tablespoon cocoa powder

1 tablespoon ground chia seed (or flax meal)

5 dried pitted dates

3/4 cup flaked coconut

2 tablespoons sweetener*

1 teaspoon cinnamon

INSTRUCTIONS

1. Heat small pot over high heat. Add cashews and enough water to cover. Boil cashews until softened, about 8 minutes.
2. Add softened cashews to food processor or bullet blender with sweetener, and process until smooth. Add water to thin if mixture is too thick or chunky. Scrape into small mixing bowl.
3. Chop dates and almonds by hand or in food processor or bullet blender. Add to cashew cream with almond butter and mix together.
4. Add cocoa powder, chia or flax meal, coconut and cinnamon, and blend.

5. Add 1 tablespoon at a time of almond butter or cocoa powder to get mixture to perfect consistency to hold together as a ball.

6. Use mini scoop or tablespoon to portion twelve servings. Roll each serving into a ball. Place balls on parchment covered half sheet pan or plate and refrigerate for about 20 minutes.

7. Serve chilled or room temperature.

*stevia, raw honey or agave nectar

Easy Paleo Baked Peaches

Prep Time: 5 minutes

Cook Time: 25 minutes

Servings: 4

INGREDIENTS

2 ripe peaches

1/4 cup walnuts

1/4 cup dried cranberries

2 tablespoons sweetener*

Juice of 1 orange

Zest of 1 orange

1 teaspoon cinnamon

1/2 teaspoon nutmeg

1/2 teaspoon ground allspice

INSTRUCTIONS

1. Preheat oven to 375 degrees F.
2. Slice peaches in half and remove pit. Place peach halves into glass or ceramic baking dish just big enough for them to fit snuggly.
3. Chop walnuts and toss with cranberries, sweetener, spices, juice and zest of orange in small bowl.
4. Fill peach halves with fruit and nut mixture. Pour excess liquid over peaches.
5. Bake in oven for about 20 - 25 minutes, until peaches are soften and lightly browned.
6. Remove from oven and let cool about 5 minutes.

7. Serve warm or room temperature.

*stevia, raw honey or agave nectar

Cave Dessert Pizza

Prep Time: 15 minutes*

Cook Time: 20 minutes

Servings: 8

INGREDIENTS

Crust

1 medium sweet potato

1 cup almond flour

2 cage-free eggs

1/4 cup tapioca flour

1 1/2 teaspoon baking powder

1 teaspoon ground cinnamon

1 teaspoon Celtic sea salt

Topping

13 oz (1 can) full-fat coconut milk

2 egg yolks

1 tablespoon tapioca powder

Juice of lemon half

Zest if lemon half

1 teaspoon vanilla

4 dried figs

1/4 cup dried apricots

1/4 cup dried cranberries

1/3 cup dried cherries

INSTRUCTIONS

1. Preheat oven to 350 degrees F. Bring medium pot of lightly salted water to a boil. Cover sheet pan with parchment paper, baking mat, or aluminum foil coated with coconut oil.

2. Peel and dice sweet potato. Add sweet potato and figs to pot and boil 5 - 10 minutes, or until soft.

3. While potatoes boil, heat small pot over medium heat. Add coconut milk, egg yolks, 1 tablespoon tapioca flour, juice and zest of half a lemon. Stir until thickened, about 5 - 10 minutes. Remove from heat and set aside.

4. Drain sweet potatoes and figs in colander. Set figs aside to cool. Add sweet potatoes to medium mixing bowl and mash with hand mixer or whisk. Add 2 eggs and beat well. Then mix in, almond flour, tapioca flour, baking powder, cinnamon and salt with wooden spoon to form dough.

5. Place dough on sheet pan and cover with parchment sheet. Press into round disc with palms, then flatten with rolling pin if desired. Remove top parchment sheet.

6. Bake crust for 20 minutes until center is firm and edges are lightly browned.

7. Chop softened figs and apricots.

8. Carefully remove crust and turn oven to broil. Evenly spread coconut lemon sauce over crust and sprinkle with dried fruit.

9. Return pizza to oven and broil for 2 minutes, just to heat toppings.

10. Remove pizza from oven. Slice and serve warm.

stevia, raw honey or agave nectar

Cave-Italy Flatbread

Prep Time: 10 minutes

Cook Time: 15 minutes

Servings: 4

INGREDIENTS

1 cup coconut flour

1/2 cup tapioca flour

1/4 cup chia seed meal (or flax meal)

2 cage-free eggs

3/4 cup water

1 teaspoon baking powder

1 teaspoon dried basil

1 teaspoon dried oregano

1/2 teaspoon ground black pepper

1/2 teaspoon Celtic sea salt

INSTRUCTIONS

1. Preheat oven to 350 degrees F. Line sheet pan with parchment paper. Prepare two additional sheets of parchment paper.

2. Whisk eggs and water in medium bowl. Set aside.

3. Combine flours, chia meal, baking powder and salt in medium bowl.

4. Pour egg mixture into flour mixture, plus spices. Mix well until dough pulls together. If dough is sticky, add 1 tablespoon of coconut flour at a time to reach proper consistency.

5. Flatten dough into basic square shape with hands on one sheet of parchment on cutting board. Cover with second sheet and use rolling pin flatten dough to about 1/8 inch thick rectangle.

6. Cut flatbread dough with pizza cutter or sharp knife into four equal pieces.

7. Gently remove top used parchment sheet and replace with fresh sheet from sheet pan. Invert sheet pan over dough and flip cutting board and sheet pan over. Replace cutting board and gently remove top used parchment sheet.

8. Use spatula to separate flatbreads. Bake in oven for 12 -15 minutes, until browned and firm. Cool and serve.

NOTE: For crisper **Flatbread**, fry flattened dough segments in oiled skillet over medium heat for about 3 minutes on each side, until puffed and browned.

Dinner Recipes

Cave Beef Sliders

Prep Time: 15 minutes

Cook Time: 25 minutes

Servings: 4

INGREDIENTS

Mini Burger Buns

1 1/2 cup raw cashews

1/3 cup coconut flour

1/4 cup almond flour

3 cage-free egg yolks

3 cage free egg whites

1/4 cup coconut oil

1/4 cup nutmilk

1 teaspoon apple cider vinegar

1 teaspoon baking soda

1 teaspoon Celtic sea salt

Filling

8 oz ground meat (beef, chicken, turkey, etc.)

1 teaspoon ground black pepper

1 teaspoon paprika

1/2 teaspoon Celtic sea salt

1/2 small onion

1 mini dill pickle (or 1/2 large dill pickle)

Organic mustard

INSTRUCTIONS

1. Preheat oven to 325 degrees F. Line sheet pan with parchment paper or coat with coconut oil.
2. Preheat oven.
3. Place cashews, egg yolks, nutmilk, coconut oil and vinegar in a food processor or bullet blender. Process until smooth. Add coconut flour, almond flour and salt. Process again until a smooth, wet dough forms.
4. Beat egg whites in medium bowl with hand mixer until stiff peaks form. Add wet dough to egg whites with and blend until combined.
5. Wet hands and shape dough into 12 mini buns, similar to burger patties. Wet hands in between each bun.
6. Place buns on prepared sheet pan and bake for 10 -15 minutes, until golden and cooked through.
7. Heat large skillet or griddle over medium-high heat.
8. Mix ground meat with spices. Form into 12 mini patties. Place burgers on hot skillet or griddle and cook about 5 minutes, or until medium-well. Flip half way through cooking.
9. Remove buns from oven and allow to cool about 5 minutes.
10. Slices bun in half. Thinly slice onion and pickle. Place hamburger on bottom half of bun. Top with onion and pickle. Add mustard to taste. Top with top bun.
11. Serve warm.

Simple Zucchini Rollatini

Prep Time: 15 minutes*

Cook Time: 25 minutes

Servings: 4

INGREDIENTS

Zucchini Pasta

1 large zucchini

Pinch Celtic sea salt

Pinch ground black pepper

Cashew Ricotta

1 cup cashews

1 1/2 cups water

2 teaspoons fresh basil

1 teaspoon ground white pepper (or black pepper)

1/2 teaspoon garlic powder

1/2 teaspoon Celtic sea salt

Pasta Sauce

6 oz (1 can) organic tomato paste

1/4 cup water

1 garlic clove

1 tablespoon oregano

2 teaspoons paprika

1 teaspoon ground black pepper

1/2 teaspoon Celtic sea salt

INSTRUCTIONS

1. *For Cashew Ricotta*, soak cashews for at least 4 hours in 1 1/2 cups water. Drain and rinse. Process with basil, white pepper, garlic powder and salt in food processor or bullet blender until smooth. Add water 1 tablespoon at a time as necessary. Set aside.

2. Preheat oven to 350 degrees F. Bring medium pot of lightly salted water to boil. Line square baking pan with parchment, or lightly coat with coconut oil.

3. For *Pasta Sauce*, process all sauce ingredients in food processor or bullet blender, then pour into small pot. Heat over medium heat and stir until warm. Remove from heat and set aside.

4. Slice zucchini into thin wide strips with sharp knife or mandolin. Blanch zucchini sheets in boiling water for about 30 seconds, just to make pliable. Remove and lay on paper towel or parchment. Sprinkle with pinch of salt and pepper.

5. Spread *Pasta Sauce* on zucchini. Place dollop of *Cashew Ricotta* toward one end of zucchini sheet. Roll up zucchini around ricotta until fully rolled.

6. Place rolled zucchini in lined baking sheet and bake for about 15 minutes, until heated through.

7. Remove from oven and serve hot.

Spicy Chicken Bite Supreme

Prep Time: 5 minutes

Cook Time: 10 minutes

Servings: 4

INGREDIENTS

8 oz boneless skinless chicken

1/2 cup almond meal

1 teaspoon flax meal

1 teaspoon paprika

1/2 teaspoon cayenne pepper

1/2 teaspoon red pepper flakes

1/2 teaspoon ground black pepper

1/2 teaspoon Celtic sea salt

1 cage-free egg

1 jalapeño pepper

2 garlic cloves

2 oz organic spicy brown mustard

Coconut oil (for cooking)

INSTRUCTIONS

1. Heat a medium skillet over medium high heat. Lightly coat pan with coconut oil.

2. Slice chicken into 1x1 inch strips. Arrange slices between 2 sheets of parchment and pound with kitchen mallet or rolling pin to flatten slightly. Place flattened pieces between two paper towels to absorb excess moisture.

3. In a shallow dish, blend almond meal, flax meal, dry spices and salt.

4. Add egg , jalapeño and peeled garlic to food processor or bullet blender. Process until fairly smooth. Pour into shallow dish.

5. Dip chicken pieces into jalapeño egg, then dredge in seasoned almond meal.

6. Carefully place coated chicken pieces into hot oil and fry about 2 minutes, until golden brown and cooked through. Turn with tongs half way through.

7. Drain cooked chicken on paper towel, then transfer to serving dish.

8. Serve hot with spicy mustard.

Bacon Quesadilla

Prep Time: 10 minutes

Cook Time: 20 minutes

Servings: 2

INGREDIENTS

Filling

8 - 12 strips nitrate-free bacon

Tortillas

2 tablespoons almond flour

1 1/2 tablespoons coconut flour

1/2 tablespoon flax meal (or ground chia seed)

1/4 cup water

2 cage-free eggs

2 tablespoons coconut oil

1/4 teaspoon baking powder

Coconut oil (for cooking)

Almond Cheese

1 cup skinless almonds*

1/4 cup water

2 tablespoons coconut oil

1 tablespoon lemon juice

1 tablespoon apple cider vinegar

1 garlic clove

1/2 teaspoon Celtic sea salt

1/4 teaspoon ground white pepper (or black pepper)

Avocado Cream
1 avocado
1/4 cup full-fat coconut cream
Small bunch cilantro
Juice of half lime

INSTRUCTIONS

1. *For *Almond Cheese*, soak almonds in 1 1/2 cups water overnight. Drain and rinse.
2. Add all *Almond Cheese* ingredients to food processor or bullet blender and process until smooth. Add a few extra tablespoons of water if necessary to achieve thick but smooth consistency. Set aside.
3. Preheat oven to 425 degrees F. Heat medium skillet over medium-high heat.
4. Chop bacon and sauté in skillet until crisp and cooked through, about 5 minutes. Remove bacon and set aside.
5. Reserve half of bacon grease. Add small amount of coconut oil to pan.
6. For *Tortillas*, whisk together eggs, coconut oil and 1/4 cup water in medium bowl. In a separate bowl, blend coconut flour, almond flour, flax or chia seed, and baking powder.
7. Whisk as you slowly pour dry into wet ingredients. If batter appears too thick to spread fairly thin in pan, add up to 4 tablespoons of water 1 tablespoon at a time.

8. Use ladle or dry measure cup to pour 1/2 of batter into hot oiled pan. Tilt pan in circular motion as you pour so batter spreads thinly.

9. Cook batter for about 2 minutes, or until slightly golden and firm. Flip tortilla with tongs or spatula and cook another 2 minutes. Remove and place on paper towel or parchment.

10. Add reserved bacon grease and small amount of coconut oil to pan. Cook remaining batter for 2 minutes on each side.

11. For *Avocado Cream*, slice avocado in half and pit. Scoop flesh into food processor with coconut cream, lime juice and cilantro. Process until smooth. Transfer to serving dish.

12. To assemble quesadilla, spread *Almond Cheese* over both tortillas. Sprinkle one tortilla with crisp bacon and top with other tortilla.

13. Place quesadilla on sheet pan or baking pan. Bake for 5 minutes.

14. Slice quesadilla with sharp knife or pizza cutter. Serve hot with *Avocado Cream*.

Easy Gyro and Avocado Tzatziki

Prep Time: 5 minutes

Cook Time: 15 minutes

Servings: 1

INGREDIENTS

Soft Baked Paleo Pita

Quick Gyro Meat

4 oz ground lamb

4 oz ground beef

1/2 small onion

1 garlic clove

1/2 teaspoon dried marjoram

1/2 teaspoon dried oregano

1/2 teaspoon dried rosemary (ground or minced)

1/2 teaspoon ground black pepper

1/2 teaspoon Celtic sea salt

1 small rib romaine lettuce

1/2 tomato

1/2 small red onion

Avocado Tzatziki

1/2 small cucumber

1/2 avocado

1 teaspoon lemon juice

1 garlic clove

Pinch Celtic sea salt

1/2 teaspoon apple cider vinegar (optional)

2 mint leaves (optional)

INSTRUCTIONS

1. Preheat oven to 350 degrees F. Cover sheet pan with parchment paper or baking mat. Heat small pot over low heat. Line small loaf pan with parchment or aluminum foil.

2. Prepare *Soft Baked Paleo Pita* and place in oven.

3. For *Quick Gyro Meat*, peel onion and garlic while pita bakes. Add onion to food processor or bullet blender and process 10 - 15 seconds. Turn onion out onto cheesecloth or paper towels. Squeeze or compress onions to remove as much liquid as possible.

4. Add drained onions back to processor with lamb, beef, garlic, herbs, salt and pepper. Process until mixture is smooth. You may need to scrape down sides of bowl.

5. Spread meat mixture into bottom of prepared loaf pan and smooth top. Place in oven and bake for 10 minutes.

6. For *Avocado Tzatziki*, peel, seed and shred or grate cucumber. Peel and mince garlic. Mince mint. Slice avocado in half scoop flesh from one half into small mixing bowl. Add cucumber, garlic, lemon juice, salt, vinegar and mint (optional). Mix well, then place in refrigerator.

7. Heat medium skillet over medium-high heat and lightly coat with coconut oil.

8. Carefully remove loaf pan and release *Quick Gyro Meat*. Peel away parchment or aluminum and use tongs and sharp knife to cut lengthwise into 1/4 inch thick slices.

9. Add meat sliced to hot oiled skillet in single layer and sear about 5 minutes, until browned and cooked through. Turn over once while cooking. Meat should be charred but not burned.

10. Remove *Soft Baked Paleo Pita* from oven and let cool about 2 minutes.

11. Peel and slice red onion. Chop lettuce. Seed and chop tomato.

12. Spread pita with *Avocado Tzatziki*. Place meat down center of pita. Add lettuce, red onions and tomatoes over meat.

13. Wrap up pita and serve immediately.

Cave Meatball Sub

Prep Time: 5 minutes

Cook Time: 20 minutes

Servings: 4

INGREDIENTS

Paleo Long Roll

Meatballs

1 lb ground meat (beef, pork, chicken, turkey, bison, or any combination)

3/4 cup almond flour

1 egg

1 garlic clove

1/2 small onion

1 teaspoon dried parsley

1 teaspoon dried oregano

1/2 teaspoon ground black pepper

1/2 teaspoon Celtic sea salt

1 tablespoon coconut oil

Tomato Sauce

1 can (8 oz) organic tomato sauce

1/4 cup water

1/2 teaspoon dried oregano

1/2 teaspoon dried basil

1/2 teaspoon ground black pepper

DIRECTIONS

1. Preheat oven to 350 degrees F. Line sheet pan with parchment paper, or lightly coat with coconut oil. Or lightly coat 6 mini loaf pans with coconut oil.

2. Prepare *Paleo Long Rolls* and place in oven.

3. While bread bakes, heat large pan over medium heat and add 1 tablespoon coconut oil.

4. For *Meatballs*, peel onion and garlic and add to food processor or blender. Pulse until finely processed, but before paste forms. Or finely mince.

5. Beat egg in large bowl. Add ground meat, almond flour, spices and salt. Mix well with hands or large wooden spoon.

6. Form 24 meatballs with scoop or tablespoon, then roll in hands. Add to hot pan and brown for 10 minutes. Turn with spatula or tongs to cook on all sides.

7. Add all *Tomato Sauce* ingredients to small pot and heat over low heat. Stir and simmer, until *Meatballs* in pan are browned.

8. Add *Meatballs* to simmering *Tomato Sauce* and increase heat to medium. Simmer another 5 minutes.

9. Remove *Paleo Long Rolls* from oven and let cool about 2 minutes.

10. Slice roll along side or split through top. Use slotted spoon to fill each roll with 6 meatballs.

11. Serve hot.

Easy Sausage and Peppers

Prep Time: 5 minutes

Cook Time: 10 minutes

Servings: 4

INGREDIENTS

4 Italian sausage links (pork, chicken, etc.)

1 white onion

1 bell pepper

INSTRUCTIONS

1. Heat large skillet over medium heat. Add 1 tablespoon coconut oil.
2. Peel onion. Stem and seed pepper. Roughly chop onion and pepper. Slice sausage into 3/4 inch slices.
3. Add sausage to hot oiled skillet and sauté about 2 minutes. Then add onion and peppers. Sauté about 8 minutes, until sausage is cooked through and browned.
4. Serve hot.

Primal Chicken Souvlaki and Paleo Tzatziki

Prep Time: 10 minutes

Cook Time: 20 minutes

Servings: 1

INGREDIENTS

Soft Baked Paleo Pita

6 oz boneless skinless chicken

2 tablespoons fresh lemon juice

1/2 teaspoon dried oregano

2 garlic cloves

1/2 teaspoon Celtic sea salt

2 teaspoons coconut oil

1 rib romaine lettuce

1/2 tomato

1/2 small white onion

Paleo Tzatziki

1/2 small cucumber

1/4 cup coconut cream (or kefir)

1 teaspoon lemon juice

1/2 teaspoon apple cider vinegar (optional, if using coconut cream)

1 garlic clove

1/4 teaspoon Celtic salt

INSTRUCTIONS

1. Preheat oven to 350 degrees F. Cover sheet pan with parchment paper or baking mat. Heat small pot over low heat.
2. Prepare *Soft Baked Paleo Pita* and place in oven.
3. While pita bakes, peel and mince garlic. Pierce chicken multiple times with fork. Then cut chicken into one inch cubes.
4. Add chicken to small mixing bowl with lemon juice, oregano, garlic, salt and 1 teaspoon coconut oil. Let chicken marinate in refrigerator for 10 minutes.
5. For *Paleo Tzatziki*, peel, seed and shred or grate cucumber. Peel and mince garlic. Add to small mixing bowl with lemon juice, coconut cream, salt and vinegar (optional). Mix well, then place in refrigerator to chill.
6. Heat small skillet or griddle over medium-high heat and add 1 teaspoon coconut oil.
7. Drain marinated chicken and add to hot oiled skillet or griddle. Grill chicken for about 4 minutes on one side, the turn over and grill for another 4 minutes, or until cooked through. Chicken should be charred but not burned.
8. Remove *Soft Baked Paleo Pita* from oven.
9. Peel and slice onion. Chop lettuce. Seed and chop tomato.
10. Spread pita with chilled *Paleo Tzatziki*. Add onion, lettuce and tomato over entire pita. Place chicken down center of pita.
11. Wrap up pita and serve immediately.

Paleo Cheese Steak "Sandwich"

Prep Time: 10 minutes*

Cook Time: 15 minutes

Servings: 4

INGREDIENTS

Paleo Long Roll

Almond Cheese

1 cup soaked skinless almonds*

1 tablespoons lemon juice

1 tablespoon apple cider vinegar

1 garlic clove

1/4 teaspoon ground black pepper

1/4 teaspoon paprika

1/2 teaspoon Celtic sea salt

1/4 cup water or 2 tablespoons coconut oil

Filling

1 lb beef steak

1 small onion

1 small bell pepper

1/2 teaspoon ground black pepper

1/2 teaspoon Celtic Sea salt

INSTRUCTIONS

1. *Soak almonds in enough water to cover overnight. Drain and rinse.

2. Preheat oven to 350 degrees F. Line sheet pan with parchment paper, or lightly coat with coconut oil. Or lightly coat 6 mini loaf pans with coconut oil.

3. Prepare *Paleo Long Rolls* and place in oven.

4. While bread bakes, heat medium skillet over medium-high heat.

5. Peel onion. Stem, vein and seed pepper. Thinly slice steak, onion and pepper.

6. Add steak to hot skillet and sauté about 1 minute. Add veggies, salt and pepper. Sauté about 5 minutes, until meat is cooked and veggies are soft and caramelized. Remove from heat.

7. Remove *Paleo Long Rolls* from oven and let cool about 2 minutes.

8. Add all *Almond Cheese* ingredients to food processor or bullet blender and process until smooth. Add 1 tablespoon water or coconut oil at a time to reach preferred consistency.

9. Slice roll along side or split through top and spread on *Almond Cheese*. Then layer on meat and veggies.

10. Serve immediately.

Crisp Spinach Salad Delight

Prep Time: 15 minutes

Cook Time: 15 minutes

Servings: 2

INGREDIENTS

Spinach Salad

4 cups spinach

2 cage-free eggs

8 slices nitrate-free bacon

1 avocado

1 small onion

1/4 cup almond flour

1/2 teaspoon ground black pepper

1/4 teaspoon paprika

1/4 teaspoon Celtic sea salt

Bacon Vinaigrette

Bacon drippings

2 tablespoons coconut oil

2 tablespoons apple cider vinegar

1 teaspoon sweetener*

2 teaspoons organic mustard

1/4 teaspoon ground black pepper

INSTRUCTIONS

1. Bring small pot of lightly salted water to boil. Heat medium skillet over medium-high heat.

2. Gently add eggs to boiling water with tongs and boil about 7 - 10 minutes. Then remove and rinse under cold water. Crack shells and remove whole egg. Set aside.

3. While eggs cook, chop bacon and add to hot pan. Sauté about 5 - 8 minutes, until crisp and cooked through. Remove bacon and drain on paper towel. Reserve bacon drippings. Add drippings to small bowl once cooled slightly.

4. Lightly coat hot pan with coconut oil.

5. Add almond flour and spiced to small mixing bowl. Peel onion and cut in half. Cut onion into half-moon slices. Toss with almond flour until well coated.

6. Add coated onions to hot oiled pan. Let crisp about 1 - 2 minutes, then turn and continue cooking another minute, until fully crisp. Remove onion crisps and set aside on paper towel to drain.

7. Rinse, dry and plate spinach. Slice avocado in half, pit, and slice in peel. Slice eggs.

8. Add bacon pieces, avocado slices, sliced eggs and onion crisp to salads.

9. Add *Bacon Vinaigrette* ingredients to small bowl with reserved bacon grease and whisk well. Pour over salads.

10. Serve immediately.

*stevia raw honey or agave nectar

Ultimate Kelp Noodle Stir-Fry

Prep Time: 10 minutes

Cook Time: 10 minutes

Servings: 2

INSTRUCTIONS

1 (12 oz) package kelp noodles

8 oz grass-fed beef

1/2 sweet onion

1 red bell pepper

1 hot chili pepper

2 cloves garlic

1 inch piece fresh ginger

1/2 teaspoon paprika

1/2 teaspoon ground black pepper

1/4 teaspoon Celtic sea salt

Small bunch fresh cilantro

1 lime

Coconut oil (for cooking)

DIRECTIONS

1. Heat large skillet or medium cast-iron wok over high heat. Drain
    and rinse kelp noodles. Add to medium bowl and soak for 5
    minutes in water and juice of 1/2 lime.

2. Stem and seed peppers. Peel onion, garlic and ginger. Dice beef
    into strips and add to medium mixing bowl. Mince chili pepper,

garlic and ginger. Add to beef with salt, pepper, paprika and 1 teaspoon coconut oil. Mix with wooden spoon to evenly coat beef.

3. Slice onion and bell pepper and add to hot skillet. Sauté about 2 minutes. Add seasoned beef to skillet and sauté another 2 minutes to brown.

4. Drain kelp noodles and add to skillet. Stir until beef is browned and cooked to about medium-well, kelp noodles are heated through, and veggies caramelize.

5. Remove skillet from heat and plate stir-fry. Chop fresh cilantro.

6. Top stir-fry with cilantro and squeeze of 1/2 lime.

7. Serve hot.

Shrimp Taco Supreme

Prep Time: 15 minutes

Cook Time: 20 minutes

Servings: 4

INGREDIENTS

Grain-Free Tortillas

Filling

12 oz medium shrimp

1/2 small red onion

1 fresh jalapeño or (2 oz pickled jalapeño)

1 garlic clove

1/2 inch piece ginger root

1/4 head cabbage (1 cup shredded)

Large bunch cilantro

1 avocado

1 tomato

2 limes

Coconut oil (for cooking)

INSTRUCTIONS

1. Heat large pan over medium-high heat and lightly coat with coconut oil.
2. Prepare *Grain-Free Tortillas*, with 4 smaller portions.
3. Keep tortillas warm and moist in oven set to WARM under damp paper towel.

4. Use clean paper towel to carefully wipe out pan. Add 1 tablespoon coconut oil to pan.

5. Peel and devein shrimp, and remove tail. Peel and mince garlic and ginger. Peel and thinly slice onion. Slice fresh jalapeños.

6. Add shrimp to pan with garlic, ginger, onion and jalapeños. Sauté about 2 minutes, then squeeze juice of 1 lime and sprinkle pinch of salt and pepper over shrimp.

7. Sauté shrimp until just cooked, about 5 minutes. Remove from heat.

8. Grate radish, shred cabbage, dice tomato. Slice avocado in half, remove pit, and slice flesh in peel. Chop cilantro.

9. Remove tortillas from oven and layer with sautéed shrimp and onions. Top with shredded cabbage, radish, tomato and avocado slices. Finish with large pinch of cilantro and squeeze of lime.

10. Fold tortillas and serve warm.

Healthy Paleo Veggie Burger

Prep Time: 5 minutes

Cook Time: 20 minutes

Servings: 4

INGREDIENTS

Paleo Soft Burger Bun

Paleo Veggie Burger

2 eggs

1/2 head cauliflower

2 medium carrots

1 small white onion

1 cup walnuts (1/2 cup ground)

1/4 cup almond flour

2 tablespoons tapioca flour

2 tablespoons ground chia seed (or flax meal)

2 cloves garlic

1 teaspoon paprika

1 teaspoon ground black pepper

1 teaspoon Celtic sea salt

Topping

1 avocado

1 heirloom tomato

1 white onion

2 ribs romaine lettuce (or preferred lettuce)

INSTRUCTIONS

1. Preheat oven to 350 degrees F. Line sheet pan with parchment paper, or lightly coat with coconut oil. Or lightly coat 6 mini round cake pans with coconut oil.

2. Prepare *Paleo Soft Burger Buns* and place in oven.

3. While bread bakes, line dish with parchment paper.

4. Add walnuts and almond four to food processor or bullet blender. Process until finely ground. Add to medium mixing bowl.

5. Peel small onion and garlic. Add to processor or blender with cauliflower and carrots. Process until finely ground. Add eggs, tapioca and chia. Process until mixture becomes thickened and has batter-like consistency.

6. Add veggie mixture and spices to mixing bowl. Mix all ingredients together with hands or wooden spoon until fully combined and uniform.

7. Form veggie mixture into 4 patties and place on parchment lined dish. Place in freezer for 10 minutes.

8. Heat medium skillet over medium-high heat and add 1 tablespoon coconut oil.

9. Peel onion. Make 4 thick slices, keeping full ring intact. Using spatula, place full rings into hot oiled pan. Sear 1 minute on each side. Set aside on paper towel to drain.

10. Reduce heat to medium and coat pan with coconut oil.

11. Remove veggie patties from freezer and place in hot oiled pan. Cook 5 minutes, then carefully flip with spatula and cook another 5 minutes.

12. Remove *Paleo Soft Burger Bun* from oven and let cool about 5 minutes.

13. Cut lettuce ribs in half. Cut tomato into 4 thick slices. Slice avocado in half, pit and slice flesh in peel.

14. Slice bun in half and place lettuce on bottom bun, followed by tomato slice. Add burger patty, then grilled onion ring. Finish with a few slices of avocado and top bun.

15. Serve immediately.

Spicy Mango Fried "Rice"

Prep Time: 10 minutes

Cook Time: 15 minutes

Servings: 4

INGREDIENTS

1 head cauliflower

8 oz boneless, skinless chicken

1 mango

1 hot chili pepper

2 scallions

2 garlic cloves

3 tablespoons pure fish sauce (or coconut aminos)

3 teaspoons sesame oil (or walnut or almond oil)

1/2 teaspoon red pepper flake

1/2 lime

Coconut oil (for cooking)

INSTRUCTIONS

1. Heat large skillet or medium cast-iron wok over high heat. Lightly coat with coconut oil.
2. Cut cauliflower into florets and add to food processor with shredding attachment to rice. Or finely mince cauliflower.
3. Peel garlic and ginger and mince. Mince chili pepper. Thinly slice scallions. Carefully peel and dice mango. Dice chicken.

4. Add diced chicken, garlic, ginger, chili pepper and red pepper flake to hot skillet or wok. Sauté until chicken is golden brown and just cooked, about 3 minutes. Remove chicken and set aside.

5. Add cauliflower to hot pan or wok. Sauté about 5 minutes, until cauliflower is golden and a bit softened.

6. Add mango and scallions and cook another 2 - 5minutes, until cauliflower is cooked through.

7. Add chicken to cauliflower and stir.

8. Remove from heat and serve hot with a squeeze of lime.

Chicken "Noodle" Soup

Prep Time: 10 minutes

Cook Time: 20 minutes

Servings: 2

INGREDIENTS

Paleo Noodles

1/2 cup almond flour

1/2 cup arrowroot powder

1/2 cup tapioca flour

1 cage-free egg

2 cage-free egg yolks

1 tablespoon coconut oil

1/2 teaspoon Celtic sea salt

Soup

8 oz skin-on chicken

1 1/2 cup chicken broth or stock

1/2 cup water

2 carrots

1 celery stalk

2 teaspoons dried thyme (4 teaspoons fresh thyme)

1/2 teaspoon black pepper

Pinch Celtic sea salt

INSTRUCTIONS

1. Heat medium pot over medium-high heat. Place chicken skin-side down in hot pot. Sear and render out fat for about 5 minutes.

2. Dice carrots and celery. Add to chicken with salt and pepper.

3. Turn chicken and brown on flesh side about 5 minutes. Stir veggies as well.

4. Add thyme, chicken stock and water, and increase heat to high. Bring soup to simmer. Adjust heat as necessary and keep at simmer or soft boil.

5. For *Paleo Noodles*, sift almond flour, tapioca flour, 1/3 cup arrow powder and salt into medium mixing bowl. Make well in the center of flour mixture and add egg and yolks. Whisk eggs into flour in circular motion with a fork until dough pulls together.

6. Dust cutting board with half of remaining arrowroot powder. Turn dough out onto cutting board and knead for 5 minutes, until smooth.

7. Add 1 tablespoon coconut oil if dough is too dry. Add 1 tablespoon almond flour at a time if dough is too moist or sticky.

8. Dust cutting board with remaining arrowroot powder. Roll dough into rectangular shape with a rolling pin to about 1/8 inch thickness. Cut pasta sheet into long strips with pizza cutter or sharp knife. Or run past through pasta machine several times until desired thickness is reached. Then use cutting attachment to cut pasta into preferred style.

9. Separate noodles a bit and place gently in simmering soup for about 3 minutes.

10. Transfer to serving dish and serve immediately.

Gazpacho and Paleo Tortilla Chips

Prep Time: 20 minutes

Cook Time: 10 minutes

Servings: 4

INGREDIENTS

Grain-Free Tortillas

Gazpacho

2 (11.5 oz) cans organic tomato juice (or 3 cups juiced tomatoes)

4 plum tomatoes

2 red bell peppers

1 red onion

1 cucumber

3 garlic cloves

1/4 cup apple cider vinegar

1/4 cup coconut oil (or 2 tablespoons coconut oil and 2 tablespoons flavorful oil [walnut, almond, sesame, etc.])

1 teaspoon cracked black pepper (or ground black pepper)

1/2 tablespoon Celtic sea salt

INSTRUCTIONS

1. Seed cucumber and tomatoes. Seed, stem and vein bell peppers. Peel onion and garlic. Dice veggies, mince garlic, and add to medium serving bowl.
2. Add tomato juice, vinegar, oil, salt and pepper, and mix well. Place in refrigerator.

3. Heat medium pan over medium-high heat and coat with coconut oil.

4. For *Paleo Tortilla Chips*, prepare *Grain-Free Tortillas*.

5. Add more coconut oil to hot pan and allow to heat up. Cut tortillas into wedges with pizza cutter or sharp knife.

6. Add tortilla wedges back to hot pan in single layer and cook about 30 seconds on each side, until golden and crisp. Drain on paper towel. Repeat with remaining tortilla wedges.

7. Transfer warm *Paleo Tortilla Chips* to serving dish. Serve immediately with chilled *Gazpacho*.

Easy Paleo Chili

Prep Time: 5 minutes

Cook Time: 20 minutes

Servings: 4

INGREDIENTS

1 lb lean grass-fed ground beef (or elk, bison, turkey or chicken)

15 oz (1 can) organic tomato sauce

6 oz (1 can) organic tomato paste

1 small onion

1 bell pepper

2 cloves garlic

2 tablespoons chili powder

1 tablespoon ground cumin

1 tablespoon smoked paprika (or paprika)

1 teaspoon Mexican oregano (or dried oregano)

1 teaspoon ground black pepper

1 teaspoon Celtic sea salt

1/2 teaspoon cayenne pepper

1 tablespoon coconut oil

Celtic sea salt, to taste

INSTRUCTIONS

1. Heat medium pot over medium-high heat. Add 1 tablespoon coconut oil.
2. Peel onion and garlic. Stem and seed bell pepper. Chop and add to food processor or bullet blender. Pulse until finely minced.

3. Add to skillet and sauté for about 1 minute. Add ground beef and spices. Brown beef for about 5 minutes. Stir with whisk to break up meat well, or wooden spoon to keep beef chunkier.

4. Add whole cans of tomato sauce and paste. Stir to combine.

5. Bring to a simmer, then reduce heat to medium and cover loosely with lid to prevent splatter. Simmer about 10 minutes. Stir occasionally.

6. Use large serving spoon or ladle to serve hot.

Seared Tuna Salad

Prep Time: 10 minutes

Cook Time: 10 minutes

Servings: 1

INGREDIENTS

1 cup spinach

1 cup arugula

1 avocado

Seared Tuna

6 oz sushi-grade tuna steak

1 tablespoon sesame oil (or coconut oil)

Juice of 1/2 lemon

1 glove garlic

1/2 inch piece fresh ginger

1 teaspoon sesame seeds

Ginger Glaze

1/2 cup pure fish sauce (or coconut aminos)

1/4 cup apple cider vinegar

Juice of 1 1/2 lemons

2 tablespoons sweetener*

1 inch piece fresh ginger

1 green onion

INSTRUCTIONS

1. For *Ginger Glaze*, peel and grate fresh ginger and slice scallion. Add to small pot with fish sauce, vinegar, sweetener and lemon juice. Heat over medium heat and bring to a simmer. Simmer 5 - 7 minutes, until slightly reduced and thickened. Stir occasionally. Once reduced, transfer to serving dish and refrigerate.

2. For *Seared Tuna*, peel and grate or mince ginger and garlic. Add to small dish with lemon juice and sesame oil and mix to combine. Roll tuna steak in marinade to coat and let sit in dish for 10 minutes in refrigerator.

3. Slice avocado in half and pit. Slice flesh in peel. Place halves together to keep avocado from browning while continuing.

4. Heat small skillet over medium-high heat. Add 1 tablespoon coconut oil.

5. Place marinated tuna in hot oiled pan and sear on each side about 1 minute, until outer flesh is just crisped but inside *is not* cooked through. About 5 minutes.

6. Remove tuna and sprinkle with sesame seeds. Cut tuna into slices.

7. Plate spinach and arugula. Fan out avocado slices over salad.

8. Top salad with *Seared Tuna*. Drizzle on chilled *Ginger Glaze* and serve immediately.

*stevia, raw honey or agave nectar

Jamaican Cave Jerk Patty

Prep Time: 20 minutes

Cook Time: 30 minutes

Servings: 4

INSTRUCTIONS

Crust

2 cups almond flour

2 cage-free eggs

3 tablespoons coconut oil

1 teaspoon curry powder

1/4 teaspoon baking soda

1/2 teaspoon Celtic sea salt

Filling

8 oz meat (ground or shredded chicken, beef or pork)

1 small onion

1 tablespoon curry powder

1 teaspoon allspice

1 teaspoon chile powder

1 teaspoon cayenne pepper

1 teaspoon red pepper flake

1/2 teaspoon garlic powder

1/2 teaspoon onion powder

1/2 teaspoon ground cinnamon

DIRECTIONS

1. For *Crust*, sift almond flour into medium mixing bowl. Add baking soda, curry powder and salt.

2. Whisk eggs in small mixing bowl, then add to flour and combine. Slowly add coconut oil until malleable dough comes together.

3. Roll in plastic wrap or wrap tightly in parchment and refrigerate for 15 minutes.

4. Preheat oven to 400 degrees. Line sheet pan with parchment or baking mat. Cover cutting board with parchment. Heat medium pan over medium heat.

5. Peel and mince onion. Add to hot pan with ground or shredded meat and spices. Sauté about 5 - 10 minutes, until beef is browned. Remove from heat and set aside.

6. Remove dough from refrigerator. Divide dough into 4 portions. Roll dough into balls and flatten on parchment covered cutting board with hands. Roll into circles about 1/8 inch thick with rolling pin.

7. Scoop equal portions of *Filling* into center of one side of dough circle. Fold bare half of dough over filled half. Press edges together, letting any trapped air escape. Crimp edges of dough together with fork. Repeat with remaining dough.

8. Arrange patties on lined sheet pan and bake 15 - 20 minutes, or until dough is golden and cooked through.

9. Serve immediately. Or allow to cool and store in air-tight container.

Primal Chicken Pot Pie

Prep Time: 15 minutes

Cook Time: 30 minutes

Servings: 4

INGREDIENTS

Filling

8 oz skin-on chicken

1 1/2 cup chicken broth

2 tablespoons tapioca flour

2 tablespoons coconut oil

2 carrots

1 celery stalk

1 green bell pepper

1 small onion

2 garlic cloves

2 teaspoons dried thyme (or 4 teaspoons fresh thyme)

1 tablespoon lemon juice

1/2 teaspoon black pepper

Pinch Celtic sea salt

Crust

1/3 cup almond flour

2 tablespoons coconut flour

3 tablespoons cold coconut oil (or cacao butter)

1 cage-free egg

3 - 4 teaspoons water

1/2 teaspoon dried thyme

1/4 teaspoon Celtic sea salt

INSTRUCTIONS

1. Preheat oven to 400 degrees F. Heat medium pot over medium heat.
2. Add two tablespoon coconut oil to hot pot. Add chicken pieces skin side down. Cook about 3 minutes, then turn with tongs and continue cooking another 3 minutes. Remove chicken and set aside.
3. Whisk coconut flour into pot until smooth. Gradually whisk in chicken broth. Simmer about 5 minutes, whisking occasionally.
4. Peel and mince garlic. Chop carrots, celery, onion and bell pepper. Add to pot with thyme, salt pepper and lemon juice.
5. Chop par-cooked chicken meat. Add back to pot and simmer for 5 minutes. Remove from heat and set aside.
6. For *Crust*, add cold coconut oil to flours, thyme and salt in small bowl. Cut fat into flour with fork until crumbly. Mix in egg and enough water to bring together tender dough.
7. Divide dough into 4 portions. Roll into balls and flatten into round disks large enough to fit over mini pie tins or ceramic ramekins with hand, then rolling pin.
8. Pour *Filling* into vessels and cover with crusts. Pinch edges of dough over edges of vessels to seal in liquid. Brush top of each pie with coconut oil, coconut milk, or egg wash and sprinkle with salt. Use knife to cut a slit in the top of each pie.
9. Bake pot pies for about 15 minutes, until crust is golden.
10. Remove from oven and allow pies to cool for 10 minutes.

11. Serve warm. Or let cool completely and serve room temperature.

Cave BBQ Pork Sandwich

Prep Time: 5 minutes

Cook Time: 15 minutes

Servings: 4

INGREDIENTS

Paleo Sandwich Bread

BBQ Pork

16 oz (1 lb) boneless pork (slow roasted or fresh)

8 oz (1 can) organic tomato sauce

1/2 small sweet onion

1 garlic clove

2 tablespoons sweetener*

1 tablespoon coconut oil

1 tablespoon apple cider vinegar

2 tablespoons paprika

1/2 teaspoon ground black pepper

1 teaspoon Celtic sea salt

INSTRUCTIONS

1. Preheat oven to 350 degrees F. Lightly coat 6 mini round cake pans with coconut oil. Heat medium skillet over medium-high heat and add 1 tablespoon coconut oil.

2. Prepare *Paleo Sandwich Bread* and place in oven.

3. While bread bakes, thinly slice and shred fresh pork, and add to hot oiled skillet. Or shred roasted pork with hands or fork and set aside.

4. Peel garlic and onion. Add to food processor or bullet blender with tomato sauce, sweetener, vinegar , salt and spice. Process until smooth.

5. Sauté fresh pork about 5 - 7 minutes, until browned, then add tomato mixture to pan. Or add tomato mixture to pan and reduce about 5 minutes, then add roasted pork.

6. Stir and simmer another 5 minutes, until sauce is reduce and fresh pork is cooked through, or roasted pork is heated through.

7. Remove *Paleo Sandwich Bread* from oven and let cool about 5 minutes. Slice and fill with *BBQ Pork*.

8. Serve warm.

*raw honey or agave nectar

Smoked Salmon Eggs Benedict

Prep Time: 15 minutes

Cook Time: 25 minutes

Servings: 4

INGREDIENTS

4 cage free eggs

6 oz smoked salmon

2 sprigs fresh dill

English Muffins

1/3 cup coconut flour

1/3 cup almond flour

2 cage-free eggs

1/4 cup almond milk (or low-fat coconut milk)

2 tablespoons coconut oil

1/2 teaspoon baking soda

1 teaspoon apple cider vinegar

Hollandaise Sauce

1/2 cup ghee or coconut oil (melted)

2 cage-free egg yolks

1/2 lemon

1/4 teaspoon Celtic sea salt

INSTRUCTIONS

1. Preheat oven to 400 degrees F. Coat 2 mini-round cake pans or 4-inch diameter ceramic ramekins with coconut oil. Bring medium pot to simmer with 1 teaspoon salt and 1 teaspoon apple cider vinegar.

2. For *English Muffins*, mix baking soda and apple cider vinegar In small bowl. Set aside and allow to froth.

3. In medium mixing bowl, beat egg whites with hand mixer or whisk until thick and frothy. Add yolks, almond and coconut flour, nut milk, and coconut oil. Mix gently.

4. Add baking soda and vinegar mixture to bowl and blend well until smooth and free of clumps.

5. Pour batter into pans or ramekins and place on sheet pan. Place in oven and bake 15 -18 minutes, until golden brown and center is firm to the touch.

6. Crack eggs into 4 separate small bowls. Coat or spray metal ladle with coconut oil. Hold ladle over simmering water and pour 1 egg into coated ladle. Slowly tilt edge of ladle into hot water, filling it gently while keeping ladle just submerged in water. Do not let egg float out of ladle or submerge ladle into water entirely. Hold and cook egg about 1 - 2 minutes, until whites are opaque and yolk is warmed but still runny. Place poached egg on paper towel to drain. Repeat with remaining eggs.

7. Remove muffins from oven. Loosen from sides of cake pans or ramekins with knife and turn out onto wire rack to cool.

8. For *Hollandaise Sauce*, add egg yolks, squeeze of lemon, and salt to food processor or high-speed blender. Processor for 30 seconds. While processor or blender is running, drizzle in melted ghee or

coconut oil very slowly. Process until all fat is added and emulsified and sauce thickens a bit, about 2 minutes.

9. Cut slightly cool *English Muffins* in half and transfer to serving dish.

10. Layer *English Muffin* halves with smoked salmon, then top with a poached egg. Pour *Hollandaise Sauce* over poached eggs, to taste. Sprinkle with pinch of salt and cracked black pepper, if preferred. Chop dill and sprinkle over eggs.

11. Serve immediately.

Half Shell Oysters

Prep Time: 15 minutes

Cook Time: 5 minutes

Servings: 2

INGREDIENTS

12 fresh whole oysters

1/2 lemon

Mignonette Sauce

1 shallot

1/3 cup Champagne vinegar or white wine vinegar (or 3 tablespoons apple cider vinegar + 1/4 cup sparkling apple cider)

1 teaspoon sweetener*

1/2 teaspoon ground black pepper

Small fresh parsley

INSTRUCTIONS

1. Have fishmonger or market personnel shuck fresh oysters to avoid damaging oyster or injuring self.
2. Place shucked oysters on serving dish. Slice lemon into wedges and place around oysters. Refrigerate until ready to serve.
3. For *Mignonette Sauce*, peel and mince shallot. Add to small pan with vinegar and sweetener and bring to boil. Cook for 1 minute, then remove pan from heat. Transfer to small serving bowl. Refrigerate until cool.

4. Chop 1 teaspoon fresh parsley and add to chilled *Mignonette Sauce* with pepper. Mix to combine.

5. Serve oysters chilled with *Mignonette Sauce* and lemon.

Almond Crusted Pan Seared Scallops

Prep Time: 15 minutes

Cook Time:10 minutes

Servings: 2

INGREDIENTS

12 large sea scallops (shelled and cleaned)

1/2 cup organic white wine (or sparkling apple cider)

1/3 cup raw almonds

1 tablespoon ground coriander

1/4 teaspoon fresh ground nutmeg

1/4 teaspoon black pepper

1/2 teaspoon Celtic sea Salt

1/2 tablespoon coconut oil

INSTRUCTIONS

1. Preheat oven to 375 degrees F.
2. Add scallops, wine and 1/4 teaspoon salt to small mixing bowl. Set aside to marinate for 10 minutes.
3. Place almonds on dry baking sheet and place in oven. Toast 7 - 8 minutes.
4. Heat medium pan over medium-high heat and add coconut oil.
5. Remove almonds from oven and add to food processor with coriander, nutmeg, 1/4 teaspoon salt and black pepper. Pulse to grind coarsely.
6. Add almond coating to shallow dish. Remove scallops from marinade and coat each side in almond mixture.

7. Place coated scallop in hot oiled pan and grill 2 - 3 minutes on each side.

8. Remove scallops and serve immediately with your favorite greens and vinaigrette.

Primal Style Marinated Baby Octopus

Prep Time: 25 minutes

Cook Time: 5 minutes

Servings: 2

INGREDIENTS

6 baby octopus

1 tablespoon chili paste

1 teaspoon coconut aminos (or apple cider vinegar)

1 teaspoon sesame oil (or walnut or almond oil)

2 tablespoons coconut oil

INSTRUCTIONS

1. Have fishmonger clean baby octopus, or remove cartilage and other entrails and gristle from octopus heads and bodies yourself.

2. Whisk together chili paste, coconut aminos and sesame oil in a small mixing bowl. Add octopus and toss to coat. Set aside to marinate for 20 minutes.

3. Heat medium pan over high heat and add coconut oil.

4. Add marinated octopus to hot oiled pan and sear about 30 seconds on each side, until just cooked through and tentacles curl. Turn halfway through cooking.

5. Transfer seared octopus to serving dish and serve hot.

Primal Shrimp Stuffed Squid Delight

Prep Time: 15 minutes

Cook Time: 25 minutes

Servings: 4

INGREDIENTS

Stuffed Squid

12 medium whole squid (calamari)

8 oz medium shrimp

2 cups baby spinach

1/3 cup almond flour

1 cage-free egg

1 tablespoon apple cider vinegar

3 garlic cloves

Small bunch fresh oregano

1/4 teaspoon crushed red pepper flakes

3/4 teaspoon Celtic sea salt

2 tablespoons coconut oil

8 wooden toothpicks

Sauce

16 oz (2 cans) organic tomato sauce

1 small onion

2 garlic cloves

1/2 cup dry white wine (or 1/3 cup sparkling apple cider + 3 tablespoons apple cider vinegar)

INSTRUCTIONS

1. Have fishmonger clean squid and peel and devein shrimp. Or clean and rinse squid and peel and devein shrimp yourself.
2. Heat medium pan over medium heat. Add coconut oil to pan.
3. Peel garlic and add to food processor or high-speed blender with shrimp and 4 squid. Pulse until coarse paste forms.
4. Add shrimp paste to medium mixing bowl. Roughly chop spinach and oregano leaves and add to bowl with egg, almond flour, vinegar, red pepper and salt. Mix to combine.
5. Stuff remaining squid bodies with stuffing. Secure closed with toothpicks.
6. Use tongs to add stuffed and secured squid to hot oiled pan. Sear for about 1 minute, then flip.
7. Peel and roughly chop onion and garlic. Add to food processor or high-speed blender with white wine. Process until onion and garlic are well broken down.
8. Pour mixture over seared squid. Add tomato sauce and gently stir to blend. Cover and simmer squid in sauce for 15 minutes.
9. Turn over stuffed squid and continue cooking uncovered another 10 minutes.
10. Remove pan from heat. Remove squid from pan and remove toothpicks from squid with tongs or forks.
11. Transfer squid to serving dish and pour sauce over.
12. Serve hot.

Oysters and Pancetta Gratin

Prep Time: 10 minutes

Cook Time: 5 minutes

Servings: 2

INGREDIENTS

6 live oysters

1 teaspoon coconut oil

2 oz pancetta

1/2 cup almonds

1/4 cup arugula

1/4 cup cherry tomatoes

1 shallot minced

2 tablespoons ghee (or coconut oil)

INSTRUCTIONS

1. Have fishmonger or market personnel shuck and clean oysters.
2. Preheat the oven to 400 F. Add coconut oil medium pan and heat over medium heat. Line sheet pan with parchment or aluminum foil.
3. Thinly slice pancetta and add to pan. Sauté 2 minutes, then remove from pan and set aside.
4. Peel and mince shallot. Chop arugula. Finely chop almonds, or add to food processor or high-speed blender and pulse to roughly grind.
5. Add pat of ghee to each oyster. Then sprinkle minced shallot, chopped arugula and crisped pancetta onto each oyster. Sprinkle with finely chopped or roughly ground almonds.

6. Place oysters on prepared sheet pan and place in oven. Bake 3 - 4 minutes, until top is golden and aromatic.

7. Remove from oven and transfer to serving dish. Slice cherry tomatoes in half and garnish dish.

8. Serve immediately.

Sage Sausage Dinner Buns

Prep Time: 10 minutes

Cook Time: 15 minutes

Servings: 8

INGREDIENTS

8 oz uncooked natural sage sausage

3/4 cup coconut flour

4 cage-free eggs

1/4 cup unsweetened applesauce

1/4 almond milk

1 teaspoon baking powder

2 tablespoons ground sage

1 tablespoon fresh basil

1 teaspoon ground white pepper (or black pepper)

1/2 teaspoon salt

INSTRUCTIONS

1. Preheat oven to 350 degrees F. Coat muffin pan with coconut oil. Heat medium skillet over medium heat.
2. Brown sausage in skillet for about 5 minutes, until half way cooked. Set aside and reserve leftover oil.
3. While sausage browns, separate eggs. In large bowl, whisk egg whites to soft peaks with hand mixer or whisk. Add yolks, applesauce and almond milk. Mix until combined.
4. Mince basil. Sift flour, baking soda and salt into egg mixture. Add pepper, sage and basil. Stir to combine.

5. Distribute par-cooked sausage evenly into each muffin pan cup. Use ice cream scoop or spoon to scoop batter on top of sausage. Fill each cup no more than 3/4 full.

6. Baste with sausage dripping before placing in oven. Bake 15 - 20 minutes, or until tops are golden brown and firm to the touch.

7. Turn out buns onto plate. Serve warm or room temperature.

NOTE: Bake in oiled square baking pan for 30 - 40 minutes for **Sage Sausage Bread**.

Paleo New Yorkshire Puddings

Prep Time: 10 minutes

Cook Time:30 minutes

Servings: 12

INSTRUCTIONS

2 cage-free eggs

1/2 cup coconut milk

1/4 cup almond flour

1/4 cup arrowroot flour

1/4 cup hazelnut flour (walnut flour or cashew flour)

1 tablespoons coconut flour

1/2 teaspoon baking soda

Pinch Celtic sea salt

Coconut oil (for cooking)

INGREDIENTS

1. Preheat oven to 400 degrees F. Line muffin pan with paper liners or pour 1/2 teaspoon coconut oil into each cup and place muffin pan in oven.
2. In medium bowl, beat eggs, milk and salt. Add flours and baking soda. Mix well. Set aside for 5 minutes while batter thickens to pudding consistency.
3. Once thickened, carefully remove hot muffin pan, and use ice cream scoop or spoon to pour batter into cups. Bake 5 minutes.

4. Reduce heat to 350 degrees F and bake 20 - 25 minutes, or until puffed and golden.

5. Turn out and plate. Serve Warm.

Tropical Guava Refresher Salad

Prep Time: 10 minutes*

Servings: 2

INGREDIENTS

2 ripe guavas

1 personal papaya (1 cup diced papaya flesh)

1 young coconut

1/2 teaspoon ground ginger (or 1/4 inch piece fresh ginger)

2 tablespoons fresh orange juice (about 1/2 orange)

INSTRUCTIONS

1. Dice guavas and add to medium mixing bowl. Peel papaya and cut in half, remove seeds and dice flesh. Remove coconut flesh from shell and dice. Add to bowl.
2. Juice orange into bowl and add ground ginger. Or peel fresh ginger and mince, then add to bowl. Toss to coat fruit evenly.
3. Transfer to serving dishes and serve immediately.
4. *Or refrigerate for 20 minutes and serve chilled.

Pastries Recipes

Almond Pizza Crust

Prep Time: 5 minutes

Cook Time: 10 minutes

Servings: 2

INGREDIENTS

1 cup almond flour

1 cage-free egg

1/2 tablespoon coconut oil

1/2 teaspoon Celtic sea salt

Pinch ground black pepper

Extra almond flour

Coconut oil (for baking)

Optional Spices:

1 teaspoon dried basil

DIRECTIONS

1. Preheat oven to 350 degrees F. Cover sheet pan with parchment paper or baking mat, or coat with coconut oil. Prepare two additional sheets of parchment and set aside on cutting board.
2. Combine all ingredients, plus *Optional Spices*, in small bowl. If too soft, add 1 tablespoon of almond flour at a time until firm dough that can hold its shape forms.

3. Form dough into ball and place on parchment covered cutting board. Press dough with palms to flatten. Then cover dough with parchment sheet and roll thin with rolling pin.

4. Carefully remove top layer of parchment from flattened dough, and place fresh parchment sheet over crust. Place sheet pan upside down over crust and careful flip thin crust onto sheet pan. Use cutting board for support to keep crust intact. Carefully peel off parchment layer (that was on the bottom and is now on top).

5. Bake crust on sheet pan in preheated oven for 5 minutes.

6. Carefully remove par baked crust and evenly spread and sprinkle with favorite sauce and toppings.

7. Return pizza to oven and bake another 5 - 10 minutes, or until toppings are heated through. Take care not to burn thin crust.

8. Turn off oven. Slice and serve hot.

9. Leave leftovers directly on oven rack (no sheet pan) to keep crust crispy.

Pizza Naan

Prep Time: 5 minutes

Cook Time: 15 minutes

Servings: 2

INGREDIENTS

1/4 cup coconut flour

2 cage-free eggs

2 tablespoons coconut oil

1/4 - 1/3 cup water

1/4 teaspoon baking powder

1/2 teaspoon Celtic sea salt

Coconut oil (for cooking)

Optional Spices:

1/2 teaspoon ground black pepper

1/2 teaspoon paprika

INSTRUCTIONS

1. Preheat oven to 350 degrees F. Heat medium skillet over medium-high heat and coat generously with coconut oil.
2. Blend flour, eggs, coconut oil, baking powder, salt, *Optional Spices* and 1/4 cup water in food processor or bullet blender. Process until smooth. Add liquid if batter is too thick, and coconut flour if too thin. You want a moderately thin batter.

3. Pour 1/2 of batter into hot oiled skillet. Cook until naan bubbles and browns. About 2 minutes. Then carefully flip naan crust with tongs and cook another 2 minutes, or until golden and firm.

4. Repeat with remaining batter. Re-oil pan as necessary. Drain hot naan on paper towel.

5. Place naan crusts on sheet pan. Evenly spread and sprinkle with favorite sauces and toppings.

6. Bake for 5 - 10 minutes, or until toppings are heated through.

7. Remove naan pizzas from oven. Slice and serve warm.

NOTE: For **Baked Primal Pizza Naan**, bake at 425 degrees F in two 9-inch round cake pans generously coated with coconut oil for 10 minutes, or until cooked through and golden.

Paleo Pizza Pita

Prep Time: 5 minutes

Cook Time: 20 minutes

Servings: 1

INGREDIENTS

1 cup tapioca flour/starch

1 cage-free egg

2 tablespoons coconut oil (or walnut oil)

1 teaspoon ground chia seed (or flax meal)

5 tablespoons water

1/2 teaspoon baking soda

1/4 teaspoon Celtic sea salt

Optional Spices:

1/2 teaspoon ground black pepper

1/2 teaspoon paprika

INSTRUCTIONS

1. Preheat oven to 375 degrees F. Line sheet pan with parchment paper. Heat small pot over low heat.
2. Mix 1/3 cup flour, chia or flax meal, water and 1 tablespoon oil in pan. Stir until mixture comes together. Remove from heat and cool in freezer.
3. In medium bowl, blend remaining flour, baking soda , salt and *Optional Spices*. Then add egg and remaining oil. Mix until combined .

4. Add cooled meal mixture to bowl. Mix to combine, then remove and knead to form dough. Form round disk, then flatten on sheet pan.

5. Bake dough for about 10 minutes in preheated oven.

6. Carefully remove crust from oven and turn over with spatula. Bake another 5 - 10 minutes, or until firm and slightly crisp.

7. Carefully remove par baked pita crust again. Evenly spread and sprinkle with favorite sauce and toppings.

8. Return pita pizza to oven and bake for 5 minutes, or until toppings are heated through.

9. Remove pizza from oven one last time. Slice with knife or pizza cutter. Serve hot.

Soft Baked Pretzel

Prep Time: 15 minutes

Cook Time: 20 minutes

Servings: 4

INGREDIENTS

1 cup coconut flour

1/2 cup tapioca flour/starch

1/2 cup coconut oil

1/2 cup water

1 cage-free egg

2 tablespoon apple cider vinegar

1/2 teaspoon baking soda

1/2 teaspoon baking powder

1/2 teaspoon Celtic sea salt

INSTRUCTIONS

1. Preheat oven to 350 degrees F. Heat medium pan over medium-high heat. Line sheet pan with parchment or baking mat.
2. Add coconut oil, water, vinegar and salt to pot. Bring to a boil and remove from heat.
3. Whisk in tapioca flour. Stir with wooden spoon or soft spatula until mixture gels and comes together.
4. Stir in baking soda and baking powder. Continue mixing for a minute. Mixture will foam and expand. Let mixture sit and cool about 5 minutes.

5. Sift in coconut flour. Mix partially, then beat in egg. Blend until combined. Excess coconut flour may sit in bottom of bowl.

6. Turn out dough onto cutting board dusted with any excess coconut flour from mixture. Knead dough for 2 minutes.

7. Cut dough into 4 equal portions. Roll out pieces into ropes and twist to form classic pretzel twist. Pinch together any crumbled dough.

8. Arrange pretzels on lined sheet pan. Brush with coconut oil or full-fat coconut milk and sprinkle with salt.

9. Place sheet pan in oven and bake about 25 minutes, until cooked through.

10. Serve immediately with organic mustard. Or allow to cool and serve room temperature.

Caveman German Chocolate Cake

Prep Time: 10 minutes

Cook Time: 15 minutes

Servings: 12

INGREDIENTS

Chocolate Cake

6 cage-free eggs

1 cup coconut flour

1/2 cup cocoa powder

1/2 cup coconut oil

1/2 cup sweetener

1/2 cup applesauce

1/2 cup dried pitted dates

1 cup water

2 teaspoons vanilla

1 teaspoon baking soda

1 teaspoon Celtic sea salt

1/4 teaspoon ground black pepper (optional)

Coconut Pecan Topping

3/4 cup flaked or shredded coconut

1/2 cup pecans

1/2 cup full-fat coconut milk

1/2 cup sweetener*

1/2 teaspoon vanilla

Pinch Celtic sea salt

INSTRUCTIONS

1. Preheat oven to 350 degrees F. Line muffin pan with paper liners or lightly coat with coconut oil. Bring 1 cup water to boil in small pan.
2. Add dried dates to boiling water for about 5 minutes.
3. For *Chocolate Cake*, sift flour, cocoa, baking soda, salt and pepper (optional) into small bowl.
4. In medium bowl, beat eggs until thick and frothy, about 5 minutes.
5. Add dates with just enough hot water to food processor or bullet blender to process into thick paste.
6. Add date paste, sweetener, applesauce, coconut oil and vanilla to eggs. Beat with hand mixer or whisk until combined.
7. Beat flour mixture into egg mixture until well combined.
8. Use ice cream scoop or spoon to pour batter into prepared muffin pan.
9. Place in oven and bake about 15 minutes, or until center is set but springy. Toothpick inserted into center should come out clean.
10. Heat small pan over medium heat.
11. For *Coconut Pecan Topping*, chop pecans and add to hot dry pan. Stir and toast pecans about 5 minutes, careful not to burn.
12. Add toasted pecans to small bowl with coconut, sweetener, coconut milk, vanilla and salt. Mix until well combined. Mixture should be thick and gooey.
13. Remove muffin pan from oven and let cool about 10 minutes.
14. Frost cakes with *Coconut Pecan Topping*.
15. Serve warm. Or allow to cool completely and serve room temperature.

NOTE: For large **German Chocolate Cake**, bake in square baking pan for 40 - 45 minutes.

* raw honey, agave nectar or maple syrup

Quick Paleo Coconut Ginger Crisps

Prep Time: 10 minutes

Cook Time: 15 minutes

Servings: 4

INGREDIENTS

1 cup coconut flour

1 cup almond flour

4 cage-free egg whites

1/2 cup sweetener

1/2 cup flaked coconut

1/4 cup coconut cream

1/4 cup organic applesauce

1/2 teaspoon baking soda

1 tablespoon ground ginger

1 teaspoon vanilla

1/2 teaspoon Celtic sea salt

INSTRUCTIONS

1. Preheat oven to 350 degrees F. Line sheet pan with parchment paper or baking mat. Prepare two additional sheets of parchment.

2. Beat egg whites with hand mixer or whisk until slightly frothy. Beat in sweetener, coconut cream and applesauce.

3. Sift in baking soda, vanilla, ginger, salt, pepper, and 1 cup of flour. Add coconut flakes and mix. Sift in remaining flour. Stir and bring dough together.

4. Form dough into rectangle and flatten with hands on extra sheet of parchment. Cover with second sheet of parchment and flatten to about 1/4 inch with rolling pin. Remove top layer of parchment.

5. Cut rectangles from dough with pizza cutter or sharp knife. Carefully transfer dough to prepared sheet pan and arrange at least 1/2 inch apart.

6. Bake for 15 minutes, or until crisp and golden brown.

7. Remove from oven and allow to cool. Serve room temperature.

*stevia, raw honey or agave nectar

Paleo Pecan Blast Shortbread Cookies

Prep Time: 5 minutes

Cook Time: 20 minutes

Servings: 12

INGREDIENTS

1 1/2 cups almond flour

1 1/2 cup pecans

1/4 cup coconut oil (or melted cacao butter)

1/4 cup sweetener*

2 teaspoons vanilla

1/4 teaspoon baking soda

1/4 teaspoon Celtic sea salt (plus extra)

INSTRUCTIONS

1. Preheat oven to 300 degrees F. Line sheet pan with parchment or baking mat.
2. Add 1 cup pecans to food processor or bullet blender and process until finely ground.
3. Add ground pecans to medium mixing bowl. Sift in almond flours, baking soda and salt.
4. Chop remaining pecans and add to small mixing bowl. Add coconut oil or melted cacao butter, sweetener and vanilla and mix to combine.
5. Pour wet mixture into dry ingredients and mix to form dough.

6. Use mini ice cream scoop or tablespoon to drop portions of dough onto prepared sheet pan. Sprinkle tops with pinch of salt if desired.
7. Place in oven and bake 20 minutes , or until lightly browned.
8. Remove from oven and let cool at least 5 minutes.
9. Serve warm or room temperature.

*raw honey, agave nectar or maple syrup

Cinnamon Raisin Cookies

Prep Time: 10 minutes

Cook Time: 20 minutes

Servings: 12

INGREDIENTS

2 cups almond flour

2 tablespoon sweetener*

1 egg

1 teaspoon vanilla

1/2 teaspoon baking powder

1/4 teaspoon Celtic sea salt

Filling

1/4 cup raisins

2 tablespoons sweetener*

2 tablespoons ground cinnamon

1/2 teaspoon ground nutmeg

1/2 teaspoon vanilla

INSTRUCTIONS

1. Preheat oven to 300 degrees F. Line sheet pan with parchment or baking mat. Prepare 2 additional sheets of parchment.

2. Add flour, egg, sweetener, vanilla, baking powder and salt to medium bowl. Blend with wooden spoon, then knead with hand to form thick dough.

3. Divide dough in half. Place half of dough in small mixing bowl. Add all *Filling* ingredients and mix until well combined.

4. Roll out each half of dough separately on parchment sheets. Roll into equal rectangles.

5. Place *Filling* rectangle on top of plain dough. Use parchment to help roll dough tightly along long edge into log.

6. Use sharp knife to cut log into 1/4 round slices. Place cookies on prepared sheet pan and bake about 10 minutes, until edges are golden brown.

7. Remove from oven and let cool about 5 minutes.

8. Serve warm. Or let cool completely and serve room temperature.

*raw honey, agave nectar or maple syrup

Cocoa Cafe Biscotti

Prep Time: 10 minutes

Cook Time: 35* minutes

Servings: 6

INGREDIENTS

1 cup almond flour

1/2 cup coconut flour

1/2 cup sweetener*

1/4 cup cocoa nibs (or organic chocolate chips)

2 tablespoons cocoa powder

1 tablespoon instant espresso (or instant coffee)

1 teaspoon vanilla

1/2 teaspoon baking soda

1/4 teaspoon Celtic sea salt

INSTRUCTIONS

1. Preheat oven to 350 degrees F. Line sheet pan with parchment or baking mat.
2. In medium mixing bowl, blend almond flour, coconut flour, cocoa powder, baking soda and salt with hand mixer or whisk.
3. Beat in sweetener, vanilla and espresso until well combined and thick, sticky dough forms. Mix in cocoa nibs or chocolate chips with wooden spoon.
4. Form dough into flattened, uniform rectangular mound about 1 - 1 1/2 inch thick on sheet pan.

5. Bake for about 15 minutes . Remove from oven and allow to cool for about 15 minutes.

6. Use a very sharp serrated knife to carefully cut biscotti log into 1/2 - 2/3 inch slices. Hold onto the mound and cut on a diagonal. If dough crumbles, stick it back together.

7. Lace slices on sides and return to oven for 15 minutes.

8. *Turn oven off and leave oven door cracked. Allow biscotti to cool and dry for at least 2 hours in oven.

9. Serve room temperature.

*raw honey, agave nectar, maple syrup, or any combination

Choco Pecan Chess Pies

Prep Time: 20 minutes

Cook Time: 25 minutes

Servings: 6

INGREDIENTS

Crust

2 cups almond flour

1 cage-free egg

2 tablespoons coconut oil

1 1/2 tablespoons cocoa powder

1/4 teaspoon Celtic sea salt

Filling

1 cup full-fat coconut milk

2 cups pecans

1 cup dried pitted dates

1/2 cups sweetener*

1/4 cup cocoa powder

2 cage-free eggs

2 cage-free egg yolks

2 tablespoons coconut oil

1 1/2 tablespoons arrowroot powder

1 teaspoon vanilla

1/4 teaspoon cinnamon

1/4 teaspoon instant coffee (optional)

INSTRUCTIONS

1. Preheat oven to 350 degrees F. Coat 6 mini pie pans with coconut oil. Bring small pot of water to boil, leaving room for dates.
2. Add dates to boiling water for about 5 minutes, until tender. Drain and set aside.
3. For *Crust*, blend almond flour, cocoa and salt in small mixing bowl. Mix in oil and egg until dough forms.
4. Press dough into pie plates with hand or wooden spoon. Bake about 10 minutes, until golden. Remove pie shells from oven and set aside.
5. For *Filling*, chop 1 cup pecans and set aside.
6. Process softened dates in food processor or bullet blender with 1/2 cup coconut milk until broken down.
7. Add date mixture to medium mixing bowl with remaining coconut milk, sweetener, cocoa, eggs, egg yolks, coconut oil, arrowroot powder, vanilla, cinnamon, and coffee (optional). Beat with hand mixer or whisk until combined and a bit lightened. Mix in chopped pecans.
8. Pour batter into mini pie crusts. Top with 1 cup whole pecans and bake for 20 - 25 minutes, until filling is set.
9. Remove pies and let cool about 20 minutes before serving.
10. Serve warm. Or refrigerate and serve cold. Also great at room temperature.

*stevia, raw honey or agave nectar

NOTE: For large **Pecan Chess Pie**, bake in 9-inch pie pan for 45 - 55 minutes, or until center is set.

Paleo Chocolate Mandarin Scones

Prep Time: 10 minutes

Cook Time: 25 minutes

Servings: 8

INGREDIENTS

2 cups almond flour

1/3 cup arrowroot powder

1/2 cup cocoa powder

Juice of 1 orange

Zest of 1 orange

1 cage-free egg

1/4 cup organic coconut oil

2 tablespoons sweetener*

2 teaspoons baking powder

1/2 teaspoon vanilla

1/2 teaspoon Celtic sea salt

INSTRUCTIONS

1. Preheat oven to 350 degrees F. Line sheet pan with parchment or baking mat.
2. Whisk together almond flour, arrowroot, cocoa, baking powder and salt in large mixing bowl.
3. Zest *then* juice orange into small mixing bowl. Add egg, sweetener and vanilla and mix with hand mixer or whisk. Beat briskly while slowly pouring in coconut oil.
4. Pour egg mixture into large bowl and mix until well combined.

5. Form dough into ball and place on prepared sheet pan . Flatten to about 1/2 inch thick circle.

6. Cut into eight wedges with pizza cutter or sharp knife. Arrange at least 1 inch apart on sheet pan and bake for 20 - 25 minutes, or until edges are browned.

7. Remove and let cool.

8. Serve room temperature.

stevia, raw honey, agave nectar or maple syrup

Cashew Crew Belgian Waffles

Prep Time: 10 minutes

Cook Time: 10 minutes

Servings: 2

INGREDIENTS

Waffles:

1 cup cashew flour (or finely ground raw cashews)

1/4 coconut flour

3 cage-free eggs, separated

1/4 cup coconut oil

4 tablespoons sweetener

1 tablespoon aluminum-free baking soda

1 teaspoon vanilla

1 pinch Celtic sea salt

1 teaspoon ground cinnamon (optional)

Topping:

1 cup fresh fruit

1/2 teaspoon vanilla

2 tablespoons water

1 tablespoon sweetener*

DIRECTIONS

1. Preheat waffle iron. Use wadded paper towel to carefully coat with coconut oil.

2. Combine flours, salt and baking soda in small bowl. In large bowl, whisk together egg yolks, oil, vanilla, plus sweetener and cinnamon (optional).

3. In separate bowl, beat egg whites to medium-stiff peaks with hand mixer. Stir flour mixture into the egg yolk mixture. Gently fold egg whites into batter.

4. Pour portion of batter onto hot waffle iron. Cook 4 - 5 minutes, until golden brown and crisp. Repeat with remain batter

5. While waffles are cooking, combine all *Topping* ingredients in small pan. Cook over stovetop until reduced and thick.

6. Top waffles with fruit compote or agave syrup (optional). Serve hot.

*stevia, raw honey, or agave nectar

Ultimate Apple Upside Down Cakes

Prep Time: 5 minutes

Cook Time: 15 minutes

Servings: 2

INGREDIENTS

1 3/4 cups almond meal

2 cage-free eggs

3/4 cup almond milk

2 tablespoons sweetener*

1 teaspoon baking powder

Juice of 1/2 lemon

1 teaspoon vanilla

1 teaspoon ground cinnamon

1 teaspoon ground nutmeg

1/4 teaspoon salt

1 tart apple

1/2 cup crushed pecans

INSTRUCTIONS

1. Heat large skillet over medium-high heat and lightly coat with coconut oil.
2. In medium bowl combine lemon juice, vanilla, cinnamon and nutmeg.
3. Peel and core apple, then slice in half length-wise. Lay halves down on flat side and slice thinly from top of apple to bottom.

Carefully toss apple slices in lemon juice and spices. Try not to break any.

4. Arrange apple slices into a circle by overlapping at the bottom and fanning out. Try to make at least 4 circles.

5. Add eggs and almond milk into leftover lemon juice and spices and whisk until combined. Add almond flour, salt and baking powder. Whisk until smooth.

6. Use oiled spatula to lift apples, keeping their arrangement, and place into hot pan. Get at least two apple arrangements into pan together. Sprinkle chopped pecans into pan around apple circles.

7. Use ladle or dry measure cup to pour 1/3 cup of batter over and around apple arrangements in skillet. Do not let pancakes touch as they spread.

8. Cook until sides of pancakes are firm and batter bubbles up a bit. About 3 - 4 minutes.

9. Flip pancakes with spatula, careful not to disturb apples. Cook for additional minute, or until cooked through. Repeat with remaining batter. Re-oil pan if necessary.

10. Pancakes will be slightly delicate, so flip and plate with care.

11. Sprinkle with cinnamon. Serve warm.

*stevia, raw honey, or agave nectar

Primal Flourless Chocolate Cake

Prep Time: 15 minutes

Cook Time: 30 minutes

Servings: 8

INGREDIENTS

16 oz organic bittersweet chocolate

1/4 cup cocoa powder

6 cage-free eggs

1 cup coconut oil

3/4 cup sweetener*

2 tablespoons water

2 teaspoons vanilla

1/4 teaspoon Celtic sea salt

INSTRUCTIONS

1. Preheat oven to 275 degrees F. Coat 2 mini springform pans with coconut oil, then dust with cocoa powder, and cover the outside base of the pans with aluminum foil. Or line muffin pan with paper liners, or leave bare and coat liners or bare pan with coconut oil and dust with cocoa powder.

2. Slowly melt chocolate and coconut oil over a double boiler, heated over medium heat. Do not boil water in bottom of double boiler. Stir frequently.

3. Remove from heat once chocolate is melted and beat in sweetener, water, vanilla, salt and any remaining cocoa powder with hand mixer or whisk.

4. Beat in eggs one at a time until thoroughly incorporated.

5. Pour batter into vessels and bake for about 25 - 30 minutes, until set. Cakes will still appear a bit glossy and wet in the middle.

6. Cool for 30 minutes, then refrigerate at least 2 hours before serving.

7. Cut springform cakes with a knife warmed until hot running water, then dried.

8. Serve chilled or room temperature.

*maple syrup, raw honey or agave nectar

Apple Dump Supreme Muffins

Prep Time: 15 minutes

Cook Time: 25 minutes

Servings: 12

INGREDIENTS

6 medium apples

1 cup almond flour

1/4 cup tapioca flour

3 cage-free eggs

1/2 cup coconut oil

1/2 cup sweetener*

2 teaspoons baking powder

2 tablespoons ground cinnamon

1 teaspoon ground nutmeg

1 teaspoon Celtic sea salt

1/2 teaspoon black pepper (or white pepper)

Juice of lemon half

INSTRUCTIONS

1. Preheat oven to 350 degrees F. Lightly coat muffin pan with coconut oil, or line with paper liners.

2. Peel, core and thinly slice apples. Add to medium bowl with 1 tablespoon cinnamon and juice of half a lemon. Evenly sprinkle on tapioca flour and carefully toss with hands to coat apples.

3. In medium mixing bowl, blend almond flour, baking powder, spices and salt. Beat in eggs, sweetener and coconut oil with hand mixer or whisk. Fold in sliced apples.

4. Scoop batter into muffin pan and bake for 20 -25 minutes, or until top is browned and firm but springy. A toothpick inserted into the center should come our moist but clean.

5. Serve warm solo, or drizzled with your favorite sweetener.

NOTE: For *Apple Dump Cake*, bake in square baking dish or Bundt pan for 40 - 50 minutes.

raw honey, agave nectar or maple syrup

Easy Pumpkin Spice Cakes

Prep Time: 5 minutes

Cook Time: 15 minutes

Servings: 12

INGREDIENTS

3/4 cup coconut flour

4 cage-free eggs

1/4 cup coconut oil

1/2 cup sweetener*

1/2 cup pumpkin purée

1 teaspoon baking soda

1 tablespoon ground cinnamon

1 tablespoon ground ginger

1 tablespoon ground nutmeg

1 tablespoon ground black pepper

1 teaspoon vanilla

1/2 teaspoon Celtic sea salt

1/4 cup pumpkin seeds

INSTRUCTIONS

1. Preheat oven to 350 degrees F. Lightly coat 4 mini cake pans or mini loaf pans with coconut oil, or line with parchment paper.
2. Sift coconut flour, baking soda, salt and spices into large mixing bowl.
3. In medium mixing bowl, beat egg whites to soft peaks with hand mixer or whisk. About 5 minutes.

4. Then beat in yolks, oil, sweetener and pumpkin purée. Mix wet ingredients into dry blend until combined.

5. Pour batter into mini cake loaf pans and sprinkle on pumpkin seeds.

6. Bake for 20 - 25 minutes, or until firm but springy in the center and browned. A toothpick inserted into the middle should come out clean.

7. Remove from oven and allow to cool for 5 minutes before serving.

8. Serve warm or room temperature.

NOTE: For large **Pumpkin Spice Cake**, oil large loaf pan or springform pan and bake 40 - 45 minutes.

raw honey, agave nectar or maple syrup

Quick Paleo Biscuits

Prep Time: 5 minutes

Cook Time: 15 minutes

Servings: 8

INGREDIENTS

2 1/2 cups fine ground almond flour

2 cage-free eggs

1/4 cup coconut oil

1 teaspoon baking soda

1/2 teaspoon Celtic sea salt

1 tablespoon sweetener*

INSTRUCTIONS

1. Preheat oven to 350 degrees F. Line sheet pan with parchment paper.
2. Combine almond flour, baking soda and salt in medium bowl.
3. Separate egg whites into separate medium bowl, and yolk into small bowl. Beat egg whites to soft peaks with hand mixer or whisk.
4. Mix yolks, oil and sweetener into whites. Mix wet ingredients into dry to form soft, solid dough.
5. Roll dough into eight (8)1-inch thick round biscuits with hands. Place on parchment covered sheet pan and bake for 12 - 15 minutes, or until golden and firm on top. Serve warm.

NOTE: Oil square baking pan, gently press in dough, cut into 9 squares, and bake for 20 - 25 minutes for break-away pan biscuits.

*stevia, raw honey or agave nectar

Classic Gingerbread

Prep Time: 5 minutes

Cook Time: 20 minutes

Servings: 8

INGREDIENTS

2 cups almond flour

2 tablespoons ground chia seed (or flax meal)

2 cage-free eggs

1/2 cup unsweetened applesauce

1/4 cup coconut oil

1/4 cup sweetener*

1 tablespoon baking powder

1 teaspoon baking soda

2 tablespoons ground ginger

1 tablespoon vanilla

1 tablespoon ground cinnamon

1 teaspoon ground black pepper

1/2 teaspoon ground cloves

1/2 teaspoon cardamom (optional)

1 oz fresh ginger juice (optional)

INSTRUCTIONS

1. Preheat oven to 350 degrees F. Coat 2 small loaf pans with coconut oil.

2. In large bowl, beat eggs until light and thickened. Add applesauce, oil, sweetener and ginger juice (optional). Beat well.

3. In medium bowl, blend all dry ingredients well. Slowly stir flour mixture into egg mixture.

4. Pour batter into loaf pans and bake for 20 - 25 minutes, or until toothpick inserted into center comes out clean.

5. Let cool slightly. Insert knife around edges and remove from pan. Serve warm or room temperature.

NOTE: Bake in large oiled loaf pan for 35 - 45 minutes for **Grain-Free Gingerbread Loaf**.

* raw honey, agave nectar, grade B maple syrup, molasses

Curry Spice Bread

Prep Time: 5 minutes

Cook Time: 20 minutes

Servings: 8

INGREDIENTS

2 cups almond flour

2 cage-free eggs

1/2 cup unsweetened applesauce

1/4 cup coconut oil

Juice of 1 lemon

Juice of 1 orange

1 teaspoon lemon zest

1 teaspoon orange zest

1 tablespoon apple cider vinegar

2 tablespoons baking powder

1 tablespoon vanilla

1 tablespoon curry powder

1 teaspoon ground cinnamon

1 teaspoon ground ginger

1 teaspoon ground white pepper (or black pepper)

1 teaspoon cardamom (optional)

1/ 4 cup pumpkin seeds (optional)

Pinch Celtic sea salt

INSTRUCTIONS

1. Preheat oven to 350 degrees F. Coat 2 small loaf pans with coconut oil.

2. Separate eggs. In large bowl, whisk egg whites to soft peaks with hand mixer or whisk. Add yolks, applesauce, oil, juices, zests and vinegar. Beat well.

3. In medium bowl, blend flour, baking powder, spices and salt. Stir flour mixture into egg mixture.

4. Pour batter into loaf pans and bake for 20 - 25 minutes, or until toothpick inserted into center comes out clean.

5. Let cool slightly. Insert knife around edges and remove from pan. Serve warm or room temperature.

NOTE: Bake in large oiled loaf pan for 35 - 45 minutes for **Citrus Curry Spice Loaf**.

stevia, raw honey or agave nectar

Banana Nut Bread Delight

Prep Time: 5 minutes

Cook Time: 20 minutes

Servings: 9

INGREDIENTS

3/4 cup of almond flour

1/4 cup of coconut flour

2 tablespoons flax meal (or ground chia seed)

2 cage-free eggs

2 overripe bananas

1/4 sweetener*

2 tablespoons coconut oil

1/4 cup walnuts

1/4 cup hazelnuts

1 tablespoon baking powder

1 tablespoon cinnamon

1 teaspoon nutmeg

1 teaspoon vanilla

1/2 teaspoon Celtic sea salt

INSTRUCTIONS

1. Preheat oven to 350 degrees F. Coat square baking pan with coconut oil.

2. In medium bowl, beat eggs, bananas, oil, flax or chia, and sweetener.

3. In separate bowl, blend flour, baking powder, salt and spices. Pour banana mixture in flour mixture and blend. Fold in nuts.

4. Pour batter into baking pan and bake for 20 - 25 minutes, or until browned and firm in the center.

5. Let cool slightly. Serve warm or room temperature.

NOTE: Bake in oiled loaf pan for 35 - 45 minutes for **Banana Nut Loaf**.

stevia, raw honey or agave nectar

Simple Squash Muffins

Prep Time: 10 minutes

Cook Time: 15 minutes

Servings: 12

INGREDIENTS

1 1/2 cups almond flour

2 tablespoons tapioca flour/starch

2 cage-free eggs

1 1/2 cups grated squash (zucchini, acorn squash, summer squash, etc.)

1/4 cup coconut oil

1/2 cup unsweetened applesauce

1/4 cup sweetener

1/2 cup walnuts

1 teaspoon baking soda

1 teaspoon baking powder

1 tablespoon ground cinnamon

1 teaspoon vanilla

1/2 teaspoon Celtic sea salt

INSTRUCTIONS

1. Preheat oven to 350 degrees F. Line muffin pan with paper liners or coconut oil.

2. Peel and chop squash. Process walnuts in food processor or bullet blender until coarsely ground. Add squash, eggs, oil, applesauce and sweetener to food processor or blender with and process until mixture is blended but slightly chunky.

3. In medium bowl, blend flours, baking soda and powder, spices and salt. Pour squash mixture into flour mixture and combine.

4. Use ice cream scoop or tablespoon to scoop batter into muffin tins, about 1/2 - 3/4 full.

5. Bake 15 - 18 minutes until muffins are golden brown and tops are firm to the touch.

6. Serve warm or room temperature.

NOTE: Bake in oiled loaf pan for 35 - 45 minutes for **Simple Squash Loaf**.

stevia, raw honey or agave nectar

Cave Kefir Rolls

Prep Time: 10 minutes*

Cook Time: 20 minutes

Servings: 8

INGREDIENTS

Starter

1 1/3 cups drained kefir milk (no kefir grains left)

1/2 cup almond flour

1/4 cup tapioca flour (or arrowroot powder)

1/2 cup warm water

2 tablespoons sweetener*

Rolls

1/2 cup almond flour

1/2 cup coconut flour

1/4 cup coconut oil

1/2 cup warm water

1 tablespoon apple cider vinegar

1 teaspoon baking soda

1 teaspoon Celtic sea salt

INSTRUCTIONS

1. *For *Starter*, add 1/2 cup water to small pot and heat over medium heat until warm. Add all *Starter* ingredients to medium mixing bowl and mix together. Cover tightly with

aluminum foil or parchment paper. Store in a warm area for 12 - 18 hours.

2. Preheat oven to 350 degrees F. Line sheet pan with parchment paper or coat with coconut oil. Or coat muffin pan with coconut oil.

3. For *Rolls*, add 1/2 cup water to small pot and heat over medium heat until warm. Sift almond flour, coconut flour, baking soda and salt into Starter. Add coconut oil and vinegar and mix to combine. Add enough warm water to form sticky dough.

4. Shape dough into rolls with hands and place on prepared sheet pan, or scoop into muffin pan.

5. Place in oven for 15 - 20 minute, until golden brown and cooked through.

6. Remove from oven and serve warm. Or allow to cool completely and serve room temperature.

* raw honey or agave nectar

Classic Everything Bagels

Prep Time:10 minutes

Cook Time: 25 minutes

Servings: 8

INGREDIENTS

2 cups almond flour

2 tablespoons coconut flour

4 cage-free eggs

1/3 cup apple cider vinegar

2 tablespoons sweetener*

2 tablespoons unsweetened applesauce

2 tablespoons ground chia seed (or flax meal)

1 tablespoon tapioca flour (or arrowroot powder)

1 teaspoon baking soda

1 teaspoon garlic powder

1 teaspoon onion powder

1 teaspoon poppy seeds

1 teaspoon sesame seeds

1 teaspoon caraway seeds (optional)

1/2 teaspoon Celtic sea salt

INSTRUCTIONS

1. Preheat oven to 350 degrees F. Lightly coat donut pan with coconut oil.

2. Add flours, chia or flax meal, baking soda and salt to food processor or high-speed blender. Process for 1 minute, until very fine.

3. Add eggs, sweetener, applesauce, vinegar, salt and spices to flour mixture. Process until fully blended, about 1 - 2 minutes.

4. Carefully scoop batter into donut pan, avoiding raised middle. Sprinkle on poppy, sesame and caraway seeds (optional).

5. Place in oven and bake for 20 - 25 minutes.

6. Remove at let cool about 5 minutes. Then remove bagels from pan.

7. Serve immediately Or let cool completely and serve room temperature.

NOTE: Bake in 8 round mini cake pans lightly coated with coconut oil if you do not have a donut pan.

stevia, raw honey or agave nectar

Cave-Cocoa Gingerbread

Prep Time: 5 minutes

Cook Time: 20 minutes

Servings: 8

INGREDIENTS

2 cups almond flour

2 tablespoons ground chia seed (or flax meal)

2 cage-free eggs

1/2 cup unsweetened applesauce

1/4 cup coconut oil

1/4 cup sweetener*

1/4 cup cocoa powder

1 tablespoon baking powder

1 teaspoon baking soda

2 tablespoons ground ginger

1 tablespoon ground cinnamon

1 teaspoon ground black pepper

1 teaspoon vanilla

1/2 teaspoon ground cloves

2 oz fresh ginger juice (optional)

INSTRUCTIONS

1. Preheat oven to 350 degrees F. Coat 2 small loaf pans with coconut oil.

2. Beat eggs in large mixing bowl with hand mixer or whisk until light and thickened, about 2 minutes. Add applesauce, oil, sweetener and ginger juice (optional). Beat well.

3. Sift all dry ingredients Into medium mixing bowl. Slowly beat flour mixture into egg mixture.

4. Pour batter into prepared loaf pans and bake for 20 - 25 minutes, or until toothpick inserted into center comes out clean.

5. Let cool at least 5 minutes. Insert knife around edges and remove brad from pan.

6. Slice and serve warm. Or let cool completely and serve room temperature.

NOTE: Bake in large oiled loaf pan for 35 - 45 minutes for **Cocoa Gingerbread Loaf**.

* raw honey, agave nectar, maple syrup, molasses

Decedent Apple Bread

Prep Time: 10 minutes

Cook Time: 20 minutes

Servings: 24

INGREDIENTS

2 cups coconut flour

1 cup almond flour

2 tablespoons tapioca flour (or arrowroot powder)

2 cage-free eggs

1 tart apple

1 sweet apple

1/2 cup unsweetened applesauce

1/4 cup coconut oil

1/4 cup sweetener*

1 tablespoon baking soda

1 tablespoon apple cider vinegar

1 teaspoon ground cinnamon

1 teaspoon ground ginger

1 teaspoon Celtic sea salt

1/2 teaspoon ground white pepper (or ground black pepper)

INSTRUCTIONS

1. Preheat oven to 375 degrees F. Line 2 muffin pans with paper liners or coat with coconut oil.

2. Peel, core and grate or dice apples, and place in small bowl. Pour vinegar and spices over apples. Toss to coat.

3. In medium bowl, whisk eggs with hand mixer or whisk until light and thickened, about 2 minutes. Add applesauce, sweetener and coconut oil. Blend until combined. Mix in apples.

4. Sift flours, baking soda and salt into apple mixture and mix until combined.

5. Use ice cream scoop or tablespoon to scoop equal portions of batter into muffin pans until 2/3 - 3/4 full.

6. Place in oven and bake for 15 - 20 minutes, or until golden brown and firm but springy to the touch.

7. Remove form oven and let cool at least 5 minutes.

8. Serve warm/ Or allow to cool completely and serve room temperature.

NOTE: Bake in oiled square baking pan for 35 - 45 minutes or two loaf pans for 45 - 55 minutes for **Primal Apple Bread Loaves**.

*stevia, raw honey or agave nectar

Honey Nut Sweet Buns

Prep Time: 10 minutes

Cook Time: 20 minutes

Servings: 8

INGREDIENTS

Dough

3 cups almond flour

3 cage-free eggs

1/2 cup dried pitted dates

1/2 cup sweetener*

1/2 cup tapioca flour (or arrowroot powder)

1/3 cup full-fat coconut milk

1 tablespoon baking powder

2 teaspoons vanilla

1/2 teaspoon ground ginger

Sweet Swirl

1/4 cup dried pitted dates

1/4 cup hot water

1/4 cup walnuts

1 teaspoon vanilla

Topping

1 cup full-fat coconut milk

1/2 cup dried pitted dates

1/2 cup sweetener*

1 cup walnuts (1/2 cup chopped)

INSTRUCTIONS

1. Preheat oven to 350 degrees F. Line muffin pan with paper liners or coat with coconut oil. Cover cutting board with parchment and coat heavily with coconut oil.

2. For *Dough*, heat coconut milk in small pan over medium heat. Whisk in tapioca or arrowroot until combined. Remove from heat.

3. Add dates, sweetener and eggs to food processor or high-speed blender. Process until thick, light mixture forms.

4. Add date mixture and tapioca mixture to medium mixing bowl. Use hand mixer or whisk to beat in chia meal, baking powder, vanilla and ginger. Beat in almond flour 1 cup at a time. Mix until dough forms.

5. Place dough on prepared parchment. Oil hands to prevent sticking and press dough into 1/2 inch thick rectangle.

6. For *Sweet Swirl*, place all ingredients in clean food processor or high-speed blender and process until finely ground. Sprinkle *Sweet Swirl* evenly over dough.

7. Roll dough into log along short edge using parchment paper. Use sharp knife or floss to slice log into rolls. Place rolls in prepared muffin pan.

8. For *Topping*, place dates, coconut milk and sweetener in clean food processor or high-speed blender and process until smooth and creamy. Pour over rolls in muffin pan. Chop walnuts (if using). Sprinkle chopped walnuts over rolls.

9. Place in oven and bake about 20 minutes, until *Topping* bubbles and browns and dough is firm.

10. Remove from oven and let cool at least 5 minutes.

11. Serve immediately. Or let cool completely and serve room temperature.

raw honey, agave nectar or maple syrup

NOTE: Bake in oiled round baking dish or cake pan for 35 minutes for **Pan Honey Nut Sticky Buns**.

Blueberry Blast Scones

Prep Time: 5 minutes

Cook Time: 25 minutes

Servings: 8

INGREDIENTS

2 cups almond flour

1/3 cup arrowroot powder (or tapioca flour)

1 cage-free egg

1/2 cup dried or frozen blueberries

1/4 cup coconut oil

2 tablespoons sweetener*

2 teaspoons baking powder

1/2 teaspoon vanilla

1/2 teaspoon Celtic sea salt

1/4 teaspoon ground cinnamon (optional)

INSTRUCTIONS

1. Preheat oven to 350 degrees F. Line sheet pan with parchment or coat with coconut oil.
2. Whisk together almond flour, arrowroot powder, baking powder, salt, vanilla and cinnamon (optional) in medium mixing bowl.
3. In small mixing bowl, beat egg, oil and sweetener with hand mixer or whisk. Add egg mixture to dry ingredients and mix until well combined.

4. Fold in blueberries. Form dough into ball and place on sheet pan . Pat down to flatten to about 1/2 inch thick circle.

5. Cut into eight wedges with pizza cutter or sharp knife. Arrange at least 1 inch apart on sheet pan and bake for 20 - 25 minutes , or until edges are golden brown.

6. Remove from oven and let cool at least 10 minutes.

7. Serve room temperature.

raw honey, agave nectar or grade B maple syrup

Pumpkin Muffins

Prep Time: 5 minutes

Cook Time: 25 minutes

Servings: 12

INGREDIENTS

1 3/4 cups coconut flour

2 cage-free eggs

15 oz (1 can) organic pumpkin puree

1 cup unsweetened applesauce

1/2 cup coconut oil

1/4 cup sweetener*

2 teaspoons baking soda

1 1/2 tablespoon ground cinnamon

1/2 teaspoon ground nutmeg

1 teaspoon Celtic sea salt

1/2 cup pumpkin seeds

INSTRUCTIONS

1. Preheat oven to 350 degrees F. Line muffin pan with paper liner or coat with coconut oil.

2. Process eggs, coconut oil, applesauce and sweetener in food processor or blender until thick and light, about 2 minutes.

3. Pour egg mixture into medium mixing bowl. Add pumpkin puree, salt and spices and mix with hand mixer or whisk.

4. Sift in coconut flour and baking soda. Mix until well combined. Stir in half of pumpkin seeds.

5. Pour batter into prepared muffin pan and sprinkle remaining pumpkin seeds over batter.
6. Place in oven and bake 20 - 25 minutes , until edges are golden and tops firm but springy.
7. Remove from oven and allow to cool 5 minutes.
8. Serve warm. Or let cool complete and serve room temperature.

*stevia, raw honey or agave nectar

Easy Cinnamon Raisin Bread

Prep Time: 5 minutes

Cook Time: 20 minutes

Servings: 12

INGREDIENTS

3/4 cup coconut flour

3/4 cup almond flour

1/4 cup ground chia seed (or flax meal)

2 cage-free eggs

1/2 cup raisins

1/2 cup coconut oil

1/2 cup unsweetened applesauce

1/4 cup sweetener*

2 tablespoons ground cinnamon

1 teaspoon baking powder

1 teaspoon Celtic sea salt

1/2 teaspoon ground black pepper (optional)

INSTRUCTIONS

1. Preheat oven to 350 degrees F. Line baking pan with parchment or coat with coconut oil.
2. In large bowl, whisk eggs with hand mixer or whisk until frothy and light. Add coconut oil, sweetener and applesauce. Blend until combined.

3. Sift coconut and almond flour, chia meal, baking powder, salt and spices into wet ingredients. Beat until smooth and well combined. Stir in raisins.

4. Pour batter into prepared baking pan.

5. Bake for 20 - 25 minutes, or until golden brown and firm to the touch.

6. Remove from oven and let cool about 5 minutes.

7. Slice and serve warm. Or allow to cool completely and serve room temperature.

NOTE: Bake in oiled loaf pan for 40 - 45 minutes for **Cinnamon Raison Bread** loaf.

stevia, raw honey or agave nectar

Paleo Cinnamon Raisin Bagels

Prep Time: 10 minutes

Cook Time: 25 minutes

Servings: 8

INGREDIENTS

2 cups almond flour

2 tablespoons coconut flour

2 tablespoons ground chia seed (or flax meal)

1 tablespoon tapioca flour (or arrowroot powder)

1 teaspoon baking soda

4 cage-free eggs

1/3 cup apple cider vinegar

1/4 cup raisins

1/4 cup sweetener*

2 tablespoons unsweetened applesauce

2 tablespoons ground cinnamon

1/2 teaspoon ground black pepper

1/2 teaspoon Celtic sea salt

INSTRUCTIONS

1. Preheat oven to 350 degrees F. Lightly coat donut pan with coconut oil.
2. Add almond, coconut and tapioca flours, chia meal, baking soda, salt and spices to food processor or high-speed blender. Process for 1 minute.

3. Add eggs, sweetener, applesauce and vinegar to flour mixture and process until fully blended, about 1 - 2 minutes. Add raisins to batter and mix until incorporated.
4. Carefully scoop batter into prepared donut pan, avoiding raised middle.
5. Place in oven and bake about 20 - 25 minutes.
6. Remove and let cool 5 minutes. Then remove from pan.
7. Slice in half and serve warm. Or let cool completely and serve room temperature.

NOTE: Bake in 8 round mini cake pans lightly coated with coconut oil if you do not have a donut pan.

stevia, raw honey, agave nectar, dried pitted dates

Paleo Chocolate Bacon Donut

Prep Time: 5 minutes

Cook Time: 20 minutes

Servings: 6

INGREDIENTS

Donuts

1 3/4 cups almond flour

1 tablespoon coconut flour

3 tablespoons cocoa powder

2 cage-free eggs

1/3 cup coconut oil

1/4 cup unsweetened applesauce

1/4 cup sweetener*

2 tablespoons nut milk (or water)

1 teaspoon baking soda

1 teaspoon vanilla

1/2 teaspoon Celtic sea salt

1/4 teaspoon ground black pepper (optional)

Topping

4 slices nitrate-free bacon

4 oz organic chocolate

2 tablespoons full-fat coconut milk

1 teaspoon cocoa powder

INSTRUCTIONS

1. Preheat oven to 350 degrees F. Lightly coat donut pan with coconut oil.

2. Add almond and coconut flours, cocoa, vanilla, baking soda, salt and pepper (optional) to food processor or high-speed blender. Process for 1 minute.

3. Add eggs, sweetener, coconut oil, applesauce, and nut milk. Process until airy batter forms, about 1 - 2 minutes.

4. Pour batter into donut pan until wells are 3/4 full.

5. Place in oven and bake for about 20 minutes, until dough is set and lightly browned.

6. For *Topping*, heat medium skillet over medium heat. Heat small pot over medium heat.

7. Chop bacon and add to hot skillet. Sauté until bacon is crisp and cooked through, about 5 minutes.

8. Add coconut milk and cocoa powder to pot and whisk. Once warmed, add chocolate and whisk.

9. Drain bacon bits on paper towel, reserving drippings. Add warm drippings to chocolate mixture. Whisk until chocolate melts and mixture emulsifies. Set bacon bits aside.

10. Remove pan from oven at let cool about 5 minutes. Then remove donuts from pan.

11. Ice donuts with chocolate sauce then sprinkle with bacon bits.

12. Transfer decorated donuts to serving dish.

13. Serve warm. Or let cool completely and serve room temperature.

NOTE: Bake in 8 mini cake pans or specialty cake pop pans lightly coated with coconut oil for fillable donuts or donut holes if you do not have a donut pan.

stevia, raw honey or agave nectar

Easy Raw Coconut Cookies

Prep Time: 35 minutes

Servings: 12

INGREDIENTS

2 cups unsweetened flaked or shredded coconut

1/2 cup raw tahini (sesame seed butter)

1/2 cup raw honey (dried pitted dates, soaked overnight)

1/2 cup raw virgin coconut oil

1 teaspoon vanilla

1/2 teaspoon Celtic sea salt

INSTRUCTIONS

1. Add tahini, honey, coconut oil, vanilla and salt to medium mixing bowl. Mix well with large wooden spoon or beat with hand mixer.
2. Add coconut and mix until well combined.
3. Use scoop or tablespoon to drop cookies onto parchment covered sheet pan. Cover and freeze at least 30 minutes, until firm.
4. Serve chilled.
5. Store leftovers in freezer.

Raw Recipes

Simple Homemade Almond Milk

Prep Time: 5 minutes*

Servings: 2

INGREDIENTS

1 cup raw almonds

4 cups water

INSTRUCTIONS

1. *Soak almonds in 1 cup water at least 6 hours, or overnight.
2. Drain soaked almonds and add to high-speed blender with 3 cups water. Process until well blended and almost smooth, about 1- 2 minutes.
3. Strain mixture through nut milk bag, cheesecloth or strainer into container.
4. Keep refrigerated up to 4 days. If milk separates, mix before use.

Simple Homemade Coconut Milk

Prep Time: 10 minutes

Servings: 2

INGREDIENTS

2 mature coconuts

3 cups water

INSTRUCTIONS

1. Remove flesh from coconuts and add to high-speed blender with 3 cups water. Process until well blended and fairly smooth, about 1-2 minutes.
2. Strain mixture through nut milk bag, cheesecloth or strainer into container.
3. Reserve pulp and set aside to dry and dehydrate, then use as coconut flour.
4. Keep refrigerated up to 4 days. If milk separates, mix before use.

NOTE: Blend additional coconut flesh with prepared coconut milk and strain for thicker coconut milk. Continue blending thickened coconut milk with additional coconut flesh until coconut cream forms. Or set thickened milk aside in refrigerator and allow fat to separate for coconut cream.

Simple Homemade Flaked Coconut Milk

Prep Time: 5 minutes*

Servings: 2

INGREDIENTS

2 cups dried coconut (unsweetened shreds or flakes)

4 cups of water

INSTRUCTIONS

1. *Soak dried coconut in 3 cups water at least 6 hours, or overnight in refrigerator.
2. Add soaked coconut and liquid to high-speed blender. Process until well blended and fairly smooth, about 1- 2 minutes. Add extra water for thinner consistency.
3. Strain mixture through nut milk bag, cheesecloth or strainer into container.
4. Reserve pulp and set aside to dry and dehydrate, then use as coconut flour.
5. Keep refrigerated up to 4 days. If milk separates, mix before use.

NOTE: Increase coconut and decrease water for thicker coconut milk. Set thickened milk aside in refrigerator and allow fat to separate for coconut cream.

Green Smoothie

Prep Time: 5 minutes*

Servings: 1

INGREDIENTS

1 cup chopped kale

1/2 cup watercress

1 banana (frozen chunks)

1 green apple

1/2 avocado

1 1/2 cups nut milk (or kefir)

2 - 4 tablespoons sweetener** (optional)

INSTRUCTIONS

1. *Peel banana, then chop and freeze.
2. Remove any stems and ribs from kale. Peel apple if preferred, then core and dice.
3. Slice avocado in half and scoop flesh of pitted half into high-speed blender. Add remaining ingredients and process until smooth, about 1 - 2 minutes.
4. Pour into large glass and serve immediately.

*Stevia, dried dates or raw honey

Nature-Blast Smoothie

Prep Time: 5 minutes

Servings: 1

INGREDIENTS

1 cup spinach

1 small zucchini (or 1/2 large)

2 celery stalks

1 cup green grapes

1 1/4 cups nut milk

2 - 4 tablespoons sweetener* (optional)

INSTRUCTIONS

1. Peel zucchini if preferred, then chop. Chop celery stalks.
2. Add all ingredients to high-speed blender. Process until smooth, about 1 - 2 minutes.
3. Pour into large glass and serve immediately.

Stevia, dried dates or raw honey

Paleo Spiced Pear Smoothie

Prep Time: 5 minutes*

Servings: 1

INGREDIENTS

2 ripe pears

1 banana (frozen chunks)

1 1/4 cups nut milk

1/2 teaspoon ground cinnamon

1/4 teaspoon ground nutmeg

1/4 teaspoon vanilla

INSTRUCTIONS

1. *Peel banana, then cut into chucks and freeze.

2. Stem and seed pears, then cut into quarters.

3. Add all ingredients to high-speed blender. Process until smooth, about 1 minute.

4. Pour into large glass and serve immediately.

Paleo Lemon Crush Refresher

Prep Time: 5 minutes

Servings: 1

INGREDIENTS

1/2 cup fresh lemon juice (about 3 lemons)

1/2 cup fresh orange juice (about 2 oranges)

1/2 cup coconut milk

1/2 cup ice

2 - 4 tablespoons sweetener*

INSTRUCTIONS

1. Juice lemons and oranges.
2. Add ice and coconut milk to high-speed blender. Pulse to crush ice.
3. Add remaining ingredients and process until smooth, about 1 minute.
4. Pour into large glass and serve immediately.

Stevia, dried dates or raw honey

Lime Cooler Crush Supreme

Prep Time: 5 minutes

Servings: 1

INGREDIENTS

1/2 cup lime juice (about 5 limes)

1 sprig fresh mint

1/2 cup thick coconut milk

2 tablespoons flaked coconut (or 1/4 cup fresh coconut)

1/2 cup ice

2 - 4 tablespoons sweetener*

1/2 teaspoon vanilla (optional)

INSTRUCTIONS

1. Remove mint leaves from stem. Juice limes.
2. Add ice and limes juice to high-speed blender. Pulse to crush ice.
3. Add remaining ingredients to high-speed blender and process until smooth, about 1 minute.
4. Pour into large glass and serve immediately.

*Stevia, dried dates or raw honey

Cocoa Chutney

Prep Time: 5 minutes*

Servings: 4

INGREDIENTS

10 oz (1 package) dried pitted dates

2 cups water

2 - 4 tablespoons raw cacao powder

1/2 teaspoon ground cinnamon

1/2 teaspoon black pepper

INSTRUCTIONS

1. *Soak dates in water over night. Drain and reserve 1/2 cup liquid.
2. Add soaked dates to medium mixing bowl. Add cacao powder and mash with large fork or potato masher for about 5 minutes, until chunky mixture forms.
3. Add soaking liquid or more cacao powder to reach desired consistency, texture and taste.
4. Add spices and mix until combined.
5. Transfer to serving dish and serve with fruits, veggies or raw breads.

Maroon Ants-On-A-Log

Prep Time: 5 minutes

Servings: 2

INGREDIENTS

3 celery stalks

2 tablespoons dried cranberries

Cashew Butter

1 cup cashews

1 dried pitted date

1 teaspoon raw virgin coconut oil

1/2 teaspoon ground cinnamon

1/4 teaspoon Celtic sea salt

INSTRUCTIONS

1. Add cashews, date, cinnamon, salt and coconut oil to food processor or bullet blender. Process until smooth. Let mixture rest between periods of processing to reach desired consistency, if necessary.
2. Cut celery stalks into thirds and fill wells with *Cashew Butter*. Place cranberries on cashew butter.
3. Serve room temperature. Or refrigerate 10 minutes and serve chilled.

Date Butter with Apples

Prep Time: 5 minutes*

Servings: 2

INGREDIENTS

1 cup dried pitted dates

2 cups water

1 teaspoon ground cinnamon

1/4 teaspoon ground ginger

1/4 teaspoon ground white pepper (or ground black pepper)

2 tart apples

INSTRUCTIONS

1. *Soak dates overnight in water. Drain and reserve soaking liquid.
2. Add soaked dates and spices to food processor or high-speed blender with 1/4 cup reserved liquid. Process on high until thick paste forms. Add more reserved liquid to thin mixture if necessary.
3. Core and slice apples
4. Transfer date butter to serving dish and serve with apple slices.

Lemon Spotted Spring Salad

Prep Time: 10 minutes*

Servings: 1

INGREDIENTS

Salad

2 cups lettuce leaves

1/2 cup dandelion leaves (optional)

2 tablespoons raw almonds (sliced or slivered)

1/4 cup fresh blueberries

Lemon Poppy Seed Dressing

3 tablespoons raw oil (coconut, walnut, almond, sesame, etc.)

2 tablespoons lemon juice

1 tablespoons sweetener*

1/4 teaspoon Celtic sea salt

1 tablespoon poppy seeds

1/4 cup raw cashews

Water

INSTRUCTIONS

1. *Soak cashews in enough water to cover for 30 minutes. Drain and rinse.

2. For *Salad*, rinse, dry and plate lettuce and dandelion leaves (optional). Sprinkle almonds and fresh blueberries over greens.

3. For *Lemon Poppy Seed Dressing*, add soaked cashews, oil, lemon juice, sweetener and salt to food processor or high-speed blender and process until smooth, about 1 - 2 minutes. Stir in poppy seeds.

4. Drizzle *Lemon Poppy Seed Dressing* over salad and serve immediately.

*stevia, raw honey or dried dates

Pecan Blast Spinach Salad

Prep Time: 10 minutes

Servings: 1

INGREDIENTS

Salad

2 cups spinach leaves

1/2 cup chopped kale leaves

4 - 5 dried apricots

3 tablespoons pecans (halves or pieces)

Honey Mustard Vinaigrette

2 tablespoons raw honey (or 2 dried dates + 2 tablespoons water)

2 tablespoons ground mustard (or mustard seed)

2 tablespoons raw apple cider vinegar

3 tablespoons raw oil (coconut, walnut, almond, sesame, etc.)

3/4 teaspoons Celtic sea salt

INSTRUCTIONS

1. For *Salad*, rinse, dry and plate spinach and kale. Chop dried apricots. Sprinkle apricots and pecans over greens.

2. For *Honey Mustard Vinaigrette*, add honey, mustard, vinegar, oil and salt to food processor or high-speed blender and process until smooth, about 1 minute.

3. Drizzle *Honey Mustard Vinaigrette* over salad and serve immediately.

Raw Blueberry Bars

Prep Time: 25 minutes

Servings: 6

INGREDIENTS

1 cup dried blueberries

1/4 cup dried pitted dates

1/2 cup raw cashews

3/4 cup raw almonds

1/4 teaspoon ground cinnamon

1/4 teaspoon vanilla

Pinch Celtic sea salt

1/3 cup warm water

1 lemon

INSTRUCTIONS

1. Soak dried blueberries and dates in warm water and lemon juice for 5 - 10 minutes.
2. Add nuts to food processor or high-speed blender. Line loaf pan with parchment paper.
3. Drain fruit and add to processor with spices and pinch of lemon zest. Process for about 1 minute, until fruit and nuts break down and the mixture sticks together when pressed.
4. Scrape mixture into prepared loaf pan and press firmly into bottom with hands or spatula.
5. Place in refrigerator and chill for 10 minutes. Remove and cut into 6 bars.

6. Serve immediately. Or store in refrigerator up to 2 weeks.

Raw Paleo Creamy Fudge

Prep Time: 10* minutes

Servings: 6

INGREDIENTS

1/4 cup raw cacao powder

3/4 cup raw almonds

1/2 cup raw hazelnuts (or cashews)

2 tablespoons raw virgin coconut oil

1/4 cup raw honey

1/4 cup hazelnuts (or walnuts)

INSTRUCTIONS

1. Line square baking dish with parchment paper.
2. Process almonds, 1/2 cup hazelnuts and coconut oil in food processor or bullet blender. Blend until fairly smooth and creamy.
3. Add nut butter, cocoa powder and honey to medium mixing bowl and mix well.
4. Chop remaining nuts.
5. *Spread mixture into parchment lined baking dish and top with chopped nuts. Refrigerate for 2 - 3 hours, until completely set.
6. Slice and serve chilled or room temperature.

Banana Cream Pie Supreme

Prep Time: 10 minutes*

Servings: 8

INGREDIENTS

Crust

1 cup raw cashews

1 cup unsweetened flaked or shredded coconut

1/2 cup dried pitted dates

1/4 teaspoon vanilla

1/4 teaspoon Celtic sea salt

Filling

2 ripe bananas

3/4 cup raw cashews

1/3 cup raw virgin coconut oil

1/4 cup raw honey

Juice of 2 lemons

1 teaspoon vanilla

Pinch teaspoon sea salt

INSTRUCTIONS

1. Place all *Crust* ingredients in food processor or high-speed blender. Process until well broken down and mixture sticks together.

2. Divide crust mixture among 4 mini pie pans. Press the crust firmly into dish your hands. Place crusts in freezer.

3. Peel bananas and add to clean food processor or blender. Juice lemons and add to processor with cashews, coconut oil, honey, vanilla and salt. Process until creamy and smooth.

4. Pour banana cream filling onto chilled crusts. Smooth tops with spatula or back of a spoon.

5. Cover pies with parchment and place in freezer for at least 30 minutes before serving.

6. Serve chilled.

7. Store leftovers in freezer.

NOTE: Press crust into single large pie pan, fill with filling and freeze for at least 3 hours for large **Raw Banana Cream Pie**.

Raw Goodness Ginger Cookies

Prep Time: 20 minutes*

Servings: 12

INGREDIENTS

3/4 cup dried apricots (1/2 cup chopped)

3/4 cup dried pitted dates (1/2 cup chopped)

1/2 cup raw macadamia nuts (frozen)

2 inch piece fresh ginger

1 teaspoon ground ginger

1/4 teaspoon ground cinnamon

1/2 cup unsweetened flakes or shredded coconut

INSTRUCTIONS

1. Place macadamia nuts in freezer for a few hours to overnight.
2. Add frozen nuts to food processor or high-speed blender. Pulse until coarsely ground.
3. Peel and finely grate fresh ginger. Add to processor with apricots, dates, ground ginger and cinnamon. Process until mixture is well broken down and sticks together.
4. Form the mixture into 12 balls and press flat. Roll cookies in coconut until well coated.
5. Cover and place in freezer for at least 10 minutes, until set up and firm.
6. Serve chilled.
7. Cover and store refrigerator or freezer until ready to serve.

Cashew Cream Chocolate Mousse

Prep Time: 5 minutes*

Servings: 2

INGREDIENTS

2 cups raw cashews

1/2 unsweetened flaked or shredded coconut

1/2 cup dried pitted dates

1/4 cup raw cacao powder

1 teaspoon vanilla

3 cups water

INSTRUCTIONS

1. *Soaked cashews and dates in 2 cups of water overnight. Separately soak coconut in 1 cup water overnight.

2. Add soaked coconut and water to high-speed blender. Process on high until smooth, about 1 minute.

3. Strain coconut mixture through nut milk bag or a few layers of cheese cloth. Squeeze out all excess liquid. Reserve coconut milk and set aside. Dry excess coconut, process until finely ground, and use as coconut flour.

4. Add drained soaked cashews and dates to clean food processor or high-speed blender with cacao powder and vanilla. Add 1/4 cup coconut milk and process on high until smooth and creamy. Add more coconut milk as necessary to reach desired consistency.

5. Pour mousse into serving dishes and serve immediately. Or freeze 15 minutes to thicken.

6. Serve room temperature or chilled.

Zucchini Salad and Primal Tomato Sauce

Prep Time: 20 minutes*

Servings: 2

INGREDIENTS

1 medium zucchini

1 tomato

5 sundried tomatoes

1 garlic clove

2 fresh basil leaves

1 tablespoon raw virgin coconut oil (or 2 tablespoons warm water)

1/4 teaspoon ground white pepper (or black pepper)

1/4 teaspoon Celtic sea salt

INSTRUCTIONS

1. Run zucchini through spiralizer, slice into long, thin shreds with knife, or use vegetable peeler to make flat, thin slices. Sprinkle with a pinch of salt and pepper, and gently toss to coat.

2. Add tomato, sundried tomatoes, peeled garlic, basil, coconut oil or warm water, and remaining salt and pepper to food processor or bullet blender. Process until sauce of desired consistency forms.

3. Transfer zucchini pasta to serving bowls. Top with tomato sauce and serve immediately.

4. Or refrigerate for 20 minutes and serve chilled.

Hot Tuna Tartare

Prep Time: 15* minutes

Servings: 4

INGREDIENTS

1 lb tuna steak (sushi grade)

1 small cucumber

1 ripe avocado

1 lime

1 garlic clove

1 hot chile pepper

2 tablespoons raw virgin coconut oil

Small bunch fresh cilantro

1 teaspoon red pepper flake

1 teaspoon Celtic sea salt

INSTRUCTIONS

1. Peel, seed and dice cucumber and avocado. Finely chop cilantro. Add to medium mixing bowl.
2. Remove seeds, stem and veins from hot pepper. Peel garlic and add to food processor or bullet blender with cayenne and hot pepper. Process until smooth paste forms. Add to bowl.
3. Dice tuna, discarding any tough white gristle. Add to bowl.
4. Squeeze on lime juice and add salt.
5. Gently toss with soft spatula or large spoon.
6. Serve immediately. Or refrigerate 20 minutes and serve chilled.

Cashew Cream Avocado Hummus

Prep Time: 5 minutes*

Servings: 4

INGREDIENTS

1 cup raw cashews

1 avocado

Juice of 1/2 lemon

2 garlic cloves

1 teaspoon ground white pepper (or black pepper)

1/2 teaspoon Celtic sea salt

INSTRUCTIONS

1. *Soak cashews in enough water to cover at least 4 hours. Drain and rinse.

2. Add soaked cashews to food processor or bullet blender with lemon juice, peeled garlic, salt and pepper. Process until smooth. Add water 1 tablespoon at a time if desired to reach thick, slightly grainy consistency.

3. Transfer cashew mixture to small mixing bowl. Cut avocado in half and remove pit. Scoop flesh into bowl and mash cashews and avocado together with fork.

4. Serve immediately. Or place in refrigerator and serve chilled.

Quick Raw Green Slaw

Prep Time: 10 minutes*

Cook Time: 20 minutes

Servings: 4

INGREDIENTS

1/2 head cabbage (2 cups shredded)

1 avocado

1 carrot

Zest of 1 lemon

Juice of 1 lemon

1 tablespoon raw honey

2 tablespoons apple cider vinegar

1 teaspoon ground white pepper (or black pepper)

1 teaspoon Celtic sea salt

INSTRUCTIONS

1. Cut avocado in half and remove pit. Scoop flesh into large mixing bowl and mash with fork.
2. Remove any tough outer leaves and core from cabbage. Shred cabbage and carrot. Add to bowl with vinegar, honey, salt and pepper. Zest *then* juice lemon, and add.
3. Toss to combine.
4. Serve immediately. Or and place in refrigerator for 20 minutes and serve chilled.

Nature's Tomato Soup

Prep Time: 5 minutes*

Servings: 2

INGREDIENTS

3 plum tomatoes (1 cup roughly chopped)

1 sundried tomato

1 clove garlic

2 large basil leaves

1/4 cup raw cashews

3/4 cup water

1/2 teaspoon Celtic sea salt

1/4 teaspoon ground white pepper (or ground black pepper)

INSTRUCTIONS

1. *Soak cashews for 4 hours, then drain and rinse, if preferred.
2. Add all ingredients to high-speed blender and process until smooth, about 2 minutes.
3. Pour into serving bowl and serve immediately.

Smoked Salmon and Green Snacks

Prep Time: 5* minutes

Servings: 2

INGREDIENTS

4 oz (1 or 1/2 package) cold-smoked salmon

1 avocado

1 stalk fresh dill

Pinch Celtic sea salt

1/2 lemon (optional)

INSTRUCTIONS

1. Slice avocado in half and remove pit. Cut into thick slices in peel then scoop out with large spoon.

2. Slice smoked salmon into long 1 inch strips. Wrap 1 salmon strips around each avocado slice. Arrange wrapped avocado on serving dish.

3. Mince fresh dill. Sprinkle dill and salt over avocado wraps and serve immediately.

4. Or squeeze juice of 1/2 lemon over avocado wraps, sprinkle on dill and salt, and refrigerate 20 minutes. Then serve chilled.

Kelp Noodle Salad and Cashew Sauce

Prep Time: 10 minutes*

Servings: 2

INGREDIENTS

1 package (12 oz) kelp noodles

1/2 lemon

1 small red bell pepper

1 small carrot

Small bunch basil leaves

Crunchy Cashew Sauce

1 cup raw cashews

1 orange

1/2 lemon

1/2 teaspoon paprika

1/2 teaspoon ground oregano

1/2 teaspoon ground black pepper

1/2 teaspoon Celtic sea salt

INSTRUCTIONS

1. *Soak 3/4 cup cashews in enough water to cover at least 4 hours. Drain and rinse.
2. Rinse and drain kelp noodles. Add to medium bowl and soak 5 minutes in warm water and juice of 1/2 lemon.
3. Cut bell pepper in half, then remove stem, seeds and veins. Thinly slice bell pepper lengthwise. Use vegetable peeler or grater to

make long, thin slices of carrot. Add veggies to medium mixing bowl.

4. For *Crunchy Cashew Sauce*, add soaked cashews, juice of lemon and orange, salt and spices to food processor or bullet. Process until very smooth.

5. Add drained kelp noodles to mixing bowl. Pour *Crunchy cashew Sauce* over veggies and kelp noodles. Chiffon basil leaves and chop remaining unsoaked cashews. Sprinkle over bowl.

6. Toss to coat. Transfer to serving dishes and serve immediately.

7. Or refrigerate for 20 minutes and serve chilled.

Craving Recipes

Sweet Cinnamon Pretzel

Prep Time: 10 minutes

Cook Time: 20 minutes

Servings: 4

INGREDIENTS

Cinnamon Pretzel

1 cup coconut flour

1/2 cup tapioca flour/starch

1/2 cup coconut oil

1/2 cup water

2 dried dates

1 cage-free egg

2 tablespoon apple cider vinegar

1/2 teaspoon baking soda

1/2 teaspoon baking powder

2 teaspoons ground cinnamon

1/2 teaspoon vanilla

1/2 teaspoon ground ginger

1/2 teaspoon Celtic sea salt

Coconut Sweet Cream

1/4 cup full-fat coconut milk

2 tablespoons sweetener

1 tablespoon lemon juice

1/2 teaspoon vanilla

INSTRUCTIONS

1. Preheat oven to 350 degrees F. Heat medium pot over medium-high heat. Line sheet pan with parchment or baking mat.

2. Add dates, coconut oil, water, vinegar and salt to food processor or bullet blender and process until smooth. Pour mixture into pot. Bring to a boil and remove from heat.

3. Whisk in tapioca flour. Stir with wooden spoon or soft spatula until mixture gels and comes together.

4. Stir in baking soda and baking powder. Continue mixing for a minute. Mixture will foam and expand. Let mixture sit and cool about 5 minutes.

5. Sift in coconut flour and spices. Mix partially, then beat in egg. Mix until combined. Excess coconut flour may sit in bottom of bowl.

6. Turn out dough onto cutting board dusted with any excess coconut flour from mixture. Knead dough for 2 minutes.

7. Cut dough into 4 equal portions. Roll out pieces into ropes and twist to form classic pretzel twist. Pinch together any crumbled dough.

8. Arrange pretzels on lined sheet pan. Brush with coconut oil or full-fat coconut milk.

9. Place sheet pan in oven and bake about 25 minutes, until cooked through.

10. For *Coconut Sweet Cream*, mix coconut milk, vanilla, sweetener and lemon juice with had mixer or whisk until thick and creamy. Transfer to serving dish.

11. Serve pretzels immediately with *Coconut Sweet Cream*. Or allow pretzels to cool and refrigerate sweet cream, and serve chilled.

stevia, raw honey or agave nectar

Choco Banana Bites

Prep Time: 10 minutes

Cook Time: 5 minutes

Servings: 1

INGREDIENTS

1 banana

2 - 4 oz organic bittersweet or semisweet chocolate

3 tablespoons chopped nuts (or flaked coconut)

DIRECTIONS

1. Heat chocolate over double boiler until melted, about 5 minutes.
2. Peel banana and cut in 1 inch slices.
3. Dip banana pieces into chocolate, or spread chocolate over tops of banana slices.
4. Sprinkle nuts or coconut over chocolate.
5. Place dipped, topped bananas in freezer for 5 minutes, or until chocolate is set.
6. Serve chilled.

NOTE: For *Frozen Chocolate Banana Bites*, leave dipped, topped banana pieces in freezer for 20 minutes, then serve.

Fruit 'N Nut Bars

Prep Time: 10 minutes

Cook Time: 10 minutes

Servings: 6

INGREDIENTS

1/4 cup dried cherries

1/2 cup dried apricots

1/4 cup dried cranberries

1/4 cup dried dates

1/3 cup warm water

1 cup cashews

1/2 teaspoon vanilla

1/2 teaspoon ground cinnamon

1/4 teaspoon ground ginger

1/4 teaspoon Celtic sea salt

INSTRUCTIONS

1. Soak dried fruit in warm water for 5 - 10 minutes. Drain and add to food processor or bullet blender with cashews, vanilla, cinnamon, ginger and salt.

2. Process until mixture forms a sticky mass, about 1 minute.

3. Transfer to loaf pan lined with parchment. Fold parchment over mixture and press firmly into bottom of pan with spatula or hand.

4. Refrigerate for 10 minutes. Remove and cut into 6 bars.

5. Serve chilled or room temperature.

Paleo Cocoa Cream Bun Delight

Prep Time: 10 minutes

Cook Time: 20 minutes

Servings: 4

INGREDIENTS

Bun

1 cup tapioca flour/starch

1/4 - 1/3 cup coconut flour

1 cage-free egg

1/2 cup warm water

1/2 cup coconut oil

1 tablespoon sweetener*

1 teaspoon apple cider vinegar

1 tablespoon cocoa powder

1/2 teaspoon cinnamon

1/2 teaspoon baking soda

1/2 teaspoon Celtic sea salt

Filling

1 cup cashews (raw or roasted)

2 tablespoons coconut cream

2 tablespoons coconut oil

2 tablespoons cocoa powder

3 tablespoons sweetener*

1/2 teaspoon cinnamon

INSTRUCTIONS

1. Preheat oven to 350 degrees F. Line sheet pan with parchment paper or coat with coconut oil. Heat medium skillet over medium-high heat.

2. For *Filling*, add cashews, coconut oil, coconut cream, cocoa powder, sweetener and cinnamon to food processor or bullet blender and process until smooth. Add 1/2 tablespoon coconut oil at a time if needed to reach desired consistency. Set aside.

3. In medium bowl, sift together tapioca flour, 1/4 cup coconut flour, cocoa powder, cinnamon, baking soda and salt. Stir in warm water and oil.

4. Whisk egg in small mixing bowl. Add sweetener and vinegar. Add egg mixture to flour mixture and mix until well combined. Add 1 tablespoon coconut flour or water at a time if needed to form soft and slightly sticky dough.

5. Divide dough into 4 portions and flatten into round disks. Dust your hand or rolling pin with extra tapioca flour to prevent sticking.

6. Scoop *Filling* into center of dough disks and pinch edges of dough together to create round, sealed ball.

7. Place buns sealed side down on sheet pan and pat down slightly. Bake 20 minutes, or until edges are golden brown and dough is cooked through.

8. Serve immediately. Or store in lidded container.

*stevia, raw honey or agave nectar

Honey Nut Bun

Prep Time: 15 minutes

Cook Time: 30 minutes

Servings: 4

INGREDIENTS

Bun

1 cup tapioca flour/starch

1/4 - 1/3 cup coconut flour

1 cage-free egg

1/2 cup warm water

1/2 cup coconut oil

1 teaspoon apple cider vinegar

1 teaspoon vanilla

1/2 teaspoon cinnamon

1/2 teaspoon baking soda

1/2 teaspoon Celtic sea salt

Filling

1 cup walnuts

1/4 cup sweetener*

2 teaspoons cinnamon

1 teaspoon ground ginger

INSTRUCTIONS

1. Preheat oven to 350 degrees F. Line sheet pan with parchment paper or coat with coconut oil. Heat medium skillet over medium-high heat.

2. For *Filling*, mix walnuts, sweetener, cinnamon and ginger in small mixing bowl. Set aside.

3. In medium bowl, sift together tapioca flour, 1/4 cup coconut flour, vanilla, cinnamon, baking soda and salt. Stir in warm water and oil.

4. Whisk egg and vinegar in small bowl. Add egg mixture to flour mixture and mix until well combined.

5. Add 1 tablespoon coconut flour or water at a time if needed to form soft and slightly sticky dough.

6. Divide dough into 4 portions and flatten into round disks. Dust your hand or rolling pin with extra tapioca flour to prevent sticking.

7. Scoop *Filling* into center of dough disks and pinch edges of dough together to create round, sealed ball.

8. Place buns sealed side down on sheet pan and pat down slightly. Bake 20 minutes, or until edges are golden brown and dough is cooked through.

9. Serve immediately. Or store in lidded container.

*stevia, raw honey or agave nectar

Chocolate Fried Pie Supreme

Prep Time: 20 minutes*

Cook Time: 20 minutes

Servings: 4

INSTRUCTIONS

Crust

2 cups almond flour

2 cage-free eggs

3 tablespoons coconut oil

1 tablespoon sweetener*

1/4 teaspoon baking soda

1 tablespoon cocoa powder

1/2 teaspoon ground cinnamon

1/2 teaspoon Celtic sea salt

Filling

1 cup cashews*

1/2 cup dried dates*

1/4 cup coconut cream

3 tablespoons cocoa powder

1 cage-free egg

1 teaspoon vanilla

1 teaspoon ground cinnamon

1 teaspoon ground nutmeg

1/2 teaspoon ground black pepper

DIRECTIONS

1. *Soak cashew and dates for at least 4 hours in 2 cups water. Drain, then add all *Filling* ingredients to food processor or bullet blender and process until smooth. Set aside.

2. For *Crust*, sift almond flour into medium mixing bowl. Add baking soda, cocoa, cinnamon and salt.

3. Whisk eggs and sweetener in small mixing bowl, then add to flour and combine. Slowly add coconut oil until formable dough comes together.

4. Roll in plastic wrap or wrap tightly in parchment and refrigerate for 15 minutes.

5. Preheat oven to 400 degrees. Line sheet pan with parchment or baking mat.

6. Remove dough from refrigerator. Divide dough into 4 portions. Roll dough into balls and flatten on parchment covered cutting board with hands. Roll into circles about 1/8 inch thick with rolling pin.

7. Scoop equal portions of *Filling* into center of one side of dough circle. Fold bare half of dough over filled half. Press edges together, letting any trapped air escape. Crimp edges of dough together with fork. Repeat with remaining dough.

8. Arrange pies on lined sheet pan and bake 15 - 20 minutes, or until dough is golden and cooked through.

9. Serve immediately.

*stevia, raw honey or agave nectar

NOTE: Heat large skillet over medium heat , add 1/4 inch coconut oil, and fry pies 2 minutes on each side for traditional *Fried Pies*.

Green Cake

Prep Time: 10 minutes

Cook Time: 30 minutes

Servings: 12

INGREDIENTS

1 1/2 cups almond flour

3 cage-free eggs

1 avocado

1 small zucchini

1 granny smith apple

1/4 - 1/2 cup sweetener*

2 tablespoons tapioca flour (or arrowroot powder)

1 teaspoon baking soda

1 teaspoon baking powder

1 teaspoon vanilla

1/4 teaspoon ground black pepper

1/2 teaspoon ground ginger

1/2 teaspoon Celtic sea salt

1/4 cup flaked coconut (optional)

INSTRUCTIONS

1. Preheat oven to 350 degrees F. Line rectangular or square baking pan with parchment or lightly coat with coconut oil.

2. Add eggs and sweetener to food processor or bullet blender. Process until mixture is thick and light in color.

3. Grate zucchini and apple and add to medium mixing bowl. Slice avocado in half, remove pit, and scoop flesh into bowl. Pour in egg mixture.

4. Sift almond flour, tapioca or arrowroot, baking soda and powder, vanilla, salt and spices into bowl. Beat with hand mixer or whisk to combine. Stir in coconut flakes (optional).

5. Pour batter into prepared baking pan and bake for about 30 minutes, until toothpick inserted into center comes out clean.

6. Remove from oven and let cool about 10 minutes.

7. Slice and serve warm. Or cool completely and serve room temperature.

*stevia, raw honey or agave nectar

Lemon Treat Coconut Cake

Prep Time: 10 minutes

Cook Time: 30 minutes

Servings: 12

INGREDIENTS

Lemon Coconut Cake

6 cage-free eggs

3/4 cup coconut flour

1 cup flaked or shredded coconut

1/2 cup unsweetened applesauce

1/2 cup lemon juice (about 5 lemons)

1/2 cup sweetener*

1/2 cup dried pitted dates

1/2 cup coconut milk

1/4 cup coconut oil

1 teaspoon vanilla

1 teaspoon baking soda

1 teaspoon baking powder

1/2 teaspoon Celtic sea salt

Lemon Coconut Icing

1/2 cup flaked or shredded coconut

1/3 cup full-fat coconut milk

1/3 cup sweetener**

Juice of 1 lemon

1/4 teaspoon vanilla

INSTRUCTIONS

1. Preheat oven to 325 degrees F. Line square baking pan with parchment or lightly coat with coconut oil.

2. Add dates, coconut milk, oil and 3 eggs to food processor or bullet blender. Process until dates break down, about 1 - 2 minutes.

3. Pour date mixture into medium bowl. Add applesauce, sweetener, lemon juice, vanilla, and remaining eggs. Beat with hand mixer or whisk until well combined.

4. Sift coconut flour, salt, baking soda and baking powder into wet ingredients. Blend until smooth. Stir in coconut.

5. Pour batter into prepared baking pan and bake for about 30 minutes, or until golden brown and toothpick inserted into center comes out clean.

6. Remove from oven and allow to cool. Place in refrigerator to speed cooling.

7. For *Lemon Coconut Icing*, beat coconut milk, sweetener, lemon juice and vanilla in small bowl until well combined. Mixture should be fairly thin and runny.

8. Coat *Lemon Coconut Cake* with *Lemon Coconut Icing*. Sprinkle on coconut.

9. Slice and serve warm. Or allow to cool completely and serve room temperature.

*stevia, raw honey or agave nectar
**raw honey, agave nectar or maple syrup

Strawberry Blondies

Prep Time: 10 minutes

Cook Time: 30 minutes

Servings: 12

INGREDIENTS

4 cage-free eggs

3/4 cup coconut flour

2 tablespoons arrowroot powder (or tapioca flour)

1 cup (1/2 pint) fresh strawberries

1/2 cup sweetener*

1/4 cup full-fat coconut milk

1/2 teaspoon baking powder

3 teaspoons vanilla

1/2 teaspoon Celtic sea salt

1/4 teaspoon ground white pepper (or black pepper)

INSTRUCTIONS

1. Preheat oven to 350 degrees F. Coat rectangular baking pan or "all-corner" specialty brownie pan with coconut oil.

2. Remove leaves and stems from strawberries. Add to food processor or bullet blender with coconut milk and process until smooth. Set aside.

3. Beat eggs in medium mixing bowl with hand mixer or whisk. Add strawberry purée, sweetener and vanilla. Mix to combine.

4. Sift coconut flour, arrowroot or tapioca, baking powder, salt and pepper (optional) into strawberry mixture. Beat until well combined.

5. Scrape batter into baking pan and smooth top with spatula.

6. Bake for 25 - 30 minutes, until center if firm and top is golden brown. Toothpick inserted into center will come out moist but mostly clean.

7. Allow to cool about 10 minutes.

8. Slice and serve warm. Or allow to cool completely and serve room temperature.

*stevia, raw honey or agave nectar

Paleo Sugar Cookies

Prep Time: 10 minutes

Cook Time: 15 minutes

Servings: 12

INGREDIENTS

1 1/2 cups almond flour

1 cup coconut flour

1/2 cup sweetener*

5 dried pitted dates

1 cage-free egg

2 teaspoons coconut oil

1 teaspoon vanilla

1/2 teaspoon baking soda

Pinch Celtic sea salt

Water

INSTRUCTIONS

1. Preheat oven to 350 degrees F. Line sheet pan with parchment paper. Bring small pot of water to boil. Add dates and boil for about 5 - 8 minutes, until softened.

2. Add dates to food processor or bullet blender and process until smooth. Add leftover water if necessary.

3. Add sweetener, egg, oil and vanilla to dates and process until smooth.

4. Add date mixture to medium bowl. Sift in almond flour, coconut flour baking soda and salt. Beat with hand mixer until combined and smooth, about 5 minutes.

5. Roll dough into a log about 3 inches in diameter. Slice into 1/4 inch thick disks.

6. Place disks on sheet pan and bake for about 8 - 10 minutes.

7. Remove from oven and cool for a few minutes.

8. Serve warm or room temperature.

stevia, raw honey or agave nectar

Primal Chocolate Cherry Brownies

Prep Time: 10 minutes

Cook Time: 25 minutes

Servings: 16

INGREDIENTS

1/2 cup fresh cherries (pitted or whole, fresh or frozen)

4 cage-free eggs

1 cup cocoa powder

2 tablespoons coconut oil

1/4 cup full-fat coconut milk

1/4 cup sweetener*

1 teaspoon vanilla

INSTRUCTIONS

1. Preheat oven to 350 degrees F. Lightly oil square baking dish or line with parchment.
2. Slice whole cherries in half and pit. Add half of cherries to food processor or bullet blender with coconut oil and process until smooth.
3. Add eggs, coconut milk, sweetener and cherry purée to medium mixing bowl and beat with hand mixer or whisk. Sift in cocoa powder and vanilla. Beat until well combined.
4. Pour batter into prepared baking pan and top with remaining cherry halves. Press cherries into batter cut side down in nice arrangement.
5. Place in oven and bake about 20 - 25 minutes, or until set.

6. Allow to cool completely.

7. Slice and serve room temperature. Or refrigerate and serve chilled.

raw honey, agave nectar or maple syrup

Mixed Berry Trifle Delight

Prep Time: 10 minutes

Cook Time: 25 minutes

Servings: 12

INGREDIENTS

Cake

1 cup almond flour

1 cup coconut flour

3/4 cup coconut milk

4 cage-free eggs

1/2 cup sweetener*

1/2 cup coconut oil

2 tablespoons vanilla

2 teaspoons baking soda

Filling

1 cup coconut cream

2 tablespoons sweetener*

1 cup strawberries

1/2 cup blueberries

1/2 cup raspberries

1/2 cup blackberries

Juice of orange half

Juice of lemon half

Zest of orange half

Zest of lemon half

1/4 cup pistachios

INSTRUCTIONS

1. Preheat oven to 350 degrees F. Line muffin pan with paper liner or coat with coconut oil.

2. In large mixing bowl, beat eggs and coconut milk until light and airy. Beat in sweetener, oil and vanilla.

3. Sift in almond flour, coconut flour and baking soda. Mix until well combined.

4. Use ice cream scoop or spoon to scoop batter into muffin pan. Fill each cup 1/2 - 2/3 full with batter.

5. Bake in for about 15 minutes, until firm but springy in the center.

6. Remove cupcakes from oven and turn out onto wire rack or plate. Allow to cool for about 10 minutes and remove paper liners.

7. Dice strawberries and add to medium bowl with blueberries, raspberries, blackberries, lemon and orange zests and juices. Toss to combine.

8. In small bowl, mixi coconut cream with 2 tablespoon sweetener.

9. Slice cupcake in half to create top and bottom. Dollop coconut cream onto bottom half, then top with a spoonful of fruit. Drain juice from spoon before adding to cake.

10. Place cupcake top on top of fruit. Press down slightly. Add another dollop of coconut cream and another spoonful of fruit. Repeat with remaining cupcakes.

11. Serve room temperature. Or chill for 30 minutes and serve.

NOTE: Bake cake in 3 round cake pans for 20 minutes, then layer with cream and berries and stack for **Mixed Berry Trifle Cake**.

stevia, raw honey or agave nectar

Carrot Cake Cookies

Prep Time: 10 minutes

Cook Time: 20 minutes

Servings: 12

INGREDIENTS

2 cups almond meal

4 large carrots (2 cups shredded)

3 cage-free eggs

1/4 cup coconut oil

1/3 cup unsweetened applesauce

1/2 cup coconut flakes

1/4 cup pitted dates

2 teaspoons vanilla

2 teaspoons ground cinnamon

1 teaspoon ground nutmeg

1 teaspoon ground ginger

INSTRUCTIONS

1. Preheat your oven to 350 Degrees F. Line sheet pan with parchment sheet or coat lightly with coconut oil.
2. Grate carrots, or process in food processor or bullet blender until finely chopped. Add to medium bowl.
3. Add eggs, oil, applesauce and dates to food processor or bullet blender. Process until thick, slightly chunky mixture forms. Pour into carrots.

4. Sift in almond meal. Then add spices and vanilla. Mix well with a wooden spoon. Stir in coconut.

5. Form 12 round balls and evenly space on sheet pan. Flatten balls with hand.

6. Bake about 20 minutes, or until firm and golden brown.

7. Remove from oven and allow to cool about 5 minutes.

8. Serve warm or room temperature.

raw honey, agave nectar or maple syrup

Chocolate Mousse

Prep Time: 5 minutes

Cook Time: 5 minutes

Servings: 2

INGREDIENTS

1 3/4 cups (about 2 cans) full-fat coconut milk

1 avocado

1/3 cup sweetener*

2 tablespoons cocoa powder

1 teaspoon vanilla

Handful cacao nibs or chapped nuts (optional)

INSTRUCTIONS

1. Process coconut milk, sweetener, cacao powder and vanilla in food processor or bullet blender until well combined.
2. Slice avocado in half and pit. Scoop flesh into mixture. Process until thick and creamy.
3. Stir in *optional* cacao nibs, nuts, etc.
4. Pour into ramekins or dessert cups and serve immediately. Or refrigerate for 1 hour to thicken.
5. Serve room temperature or chilled.

* raw honey, agave nectar or maple syrup

Paleo Plain Vanilla Pudding

Prep Time: 5 minutes

Cook Time: 10 minutes

Servings: 2

INGREDIENTS

13 oz (1 can) coconut milk

2 cage-free egg yolks

3 tablespoons sweetener*

2 tablespoons cacao butter

1 tablespoon vanilla

INSTRUCTIONS

1. Add coconut milk, sweetener and cacao butter to small pot and place over medium heat. Bring to a simmer, stirring periodically. Add vanilla.

2. In small mixing bowl, whisk 1 tablespoon hot coconut milk into egg yolks. Add second tablespoon. Slowly whisk in 1/4 cup of hot liquid, then add yolk mixture back to hot coconut milk.

3. Whisk custard constantly until thickened, about 5 minutes. Do not let pudding burn.

4. Pour hot pudding into ramekins or dessert cups and refrigerate at least 1 hour.

5. Once chilled, serve immediately. Or remove from fridge, and allow to warm up about 10 minutes and serve room temperature.

raw honey or agave nectar

Baked Donut

Prep Time: 5 minutes

Cook Time: 20 minutes

Servings: 6

INGREDIENTS

Donuts

1 3/4 cups almond flour

1 tablespoon coconut flour

2 cage-free eggs

1/3 cup coconut oil

1/4 cup unsweetened applesauce

1/4 cup sweetener*

2 tablespoons nut milk

2 teaspoons vanilla

3/4 teaspoon baking soda

1/2 teaspoon Celtic sea salt

Topping

1/2 cup flaked or shredded coconut

1/4 cup full-fat coconut milk

2 tablespoon sweetener

1/4 teaspoon vanilla

INSTRUCTIONS

1. Preheat oven to 350 degreesF. Lightly coat donut pan with coconut oil.

2. Add almond and coconut flours, baking soda and salt to food processor or high-speed blender. Process for 1 minute.

3. Add eggs, sweetener, coconut oil, applesauce, nut milk and vanilla. Process until light, thick batter forms, about 1 - 2 minutes.

4. Pour batter into donut pan until wells are 3/4 full.

5. Place in oven and bake for about 20 minutes, until dough isset and lightly browned.

6. For *Topping*, combine coconut milk, sweetener and vanilla in small mixing bowl.

7. Remove pan from oven at let cool about 5 minutes. Then remove donuts from pan.

8. Dip donuts in coconut icing then sprinkle with flaked or shredded coconut.

9. Transfer decorated donuts to serving dish.

10. Serve warm. Or let cool completely and serve room temperature.

NOTE: Bake in 8 mini cake pans or specialty cake pop pans lightly coated with coconut oil for fillable donuts or donut holes if you do not have a donut pan.

stevia, raw honey or agave nectar

Paleo Avocado Banana Bread

Prep Time: 5 minutes

Cook Time: 25 minutes

Servings: 9

INGREDIENTS

3/4 cup almond flour

1/4 cup coconut flour

2 tablespoons flax meal (or ground chia seed)

2 cage-free eggs

1 large overripe banana

1 avocado

1/4 cup sweetener*

2 tablespoons coconut oil

1 tablespoon baking powder

1 tablespoon cinnamon

1 teaspoon ground ginger

1 teaspoon vanilla

1/2 teaspoon ground black pepper

1/2 teaspoon Celtic sea salt

1/2 cup organic banana chips (optional)

INSTRUCTIONS

1. Preheat oven to 350 degrees F. Coat square baking pan with coconut oil.
2. Slice avocado in half. Remove pit and scoop flesh into medium mixing bowl. Peel banana and add to bowl with eggs,

sweetener, and flax or chia meal. Beat with hand mixer or whisk until well blended.

3. Sift flour, baking powder, salt and spices Into banana mixture. Mix until combined. Roughly chop banana chips and fold into batter (optional).

4. Pour batter into baking pan and bake for 20 - 25 minutes, or until browned and firm in the center.

5. Remove from oven and let cool at least 5 minutes.

6. Slice and serve warm. Or allow to cool completely and serve room temperature.

NOTE: Bake in oiled loaf pan for 35 - 45 minutes for **Avocado Banana Loaf**.

stevia, raw honey or agave nectar

Paleo Peach Cobbler

Prep Time: 5 minutes

Cook Time: 20 minutes

Servings: 8

INGREDIENTS

4 ripe peaches

1 cup almond flour

1/4 cup coconut oil

1/4 cup unsalted almond butter (or whole almonds)

1/4 cup dried pitted dates

2 teaspoons vanilla

2 teaspoons cinnamon

1/2 teaspoon Celtic sea salt

1 teaspoon tapioca flour or arrowroot powder (optional)

INSTRUCTIONS

1. Preheat oven to 350 degrees F. Lightly coat sides of baking dish with coconut oil.

2. Slice peaches in half and twist to release from pit. Remove pit and dice or slice peaches. Gently toss with tapioca or arrowroot in medium mixing bowl (optional).

3. Spread peaches evenly across bottom of baking dish. Sprinkle with 1 teaspoon cinnamon. Set aside.

4. Add dates, coconut oil and whole almonds (if using) to food processor or high-speed blender. Pulse until dates (and almonds) are coarsely ground. Add to medium mixing bowl with almond

flour, almond butter (if using), vanilla, remaining cinnamon and salt. Blend until crumbly mixture resembling moist graham cracker crust forms. Add coconut oil, almond butter or almond flour 1 tablespoon at a time to reach desired consistency.

5. Sprinkle crumble evenly over peaches.

6. Place in oven and bake 15 - 20 minutes, or until crumble is golden brown and crisp.

7. Remove from oven and let cool 5 minutes.

8. Scoop or slice and serve warm. Or let cool completely and serve room temperature.

Primal Berry Treat Tart

Prep Time: 20 minutes

Cook Time: 25 minutes

Servings: 4

INGREDIENTS

Tart Shell

2 cups almond flour

1 egg

2 tablespoons coconut oil

1/2 teaspoon vanilla

1/2 teaspoon Celtic sea salt

Filling

1/2 cup coconut cream (settled from1 can full-fat coconut milk)

1/4 - 1/2 cup sweetener*

1/2 teaspoon vanilla

1/4 cup fresh blueberries

1/4 cup fresh sliced strawberries

1/4 cup fresh blackberries

1/4 cup fresh raspberries

INSTRUCTIONS

1. Preheat oven to 350 degrees F. Coat four 4-inch tart pans or pie plates with coconut oil.

2. For *Tart Shell*, add almond flour, salt and vanilla to food processor or high-speed blender and process about 30 seconds.

3. Add coconut oil and egg, and process until dough comes together.

4. Press dough into prepared pans and place in oven. Bake 8 - 10 minutes, or until golden brown. Remove pie shells from oven and set aside. Refrigerate to speed cooling.

5. For *Filling*, beat coconut cream, sweetener and vanilla with hand mixer or whisk in medium mixing bowl until thickened, about 2 minutes.

6. Pour cream mixture into *Tart Shells*. Top with fresh berries.

7. Serve immediately. Or refrigerate 20 minutes and serve chilled.

stevia, raw honey or agave nectar

NOTE: Bake crust in 9-inch tart pan for 12 - 15 minutes and fill for large **Berry Tart**.

Strawberry Sweet Cake

Prep Time: 15 minutes

Cook Time: 30 minutes

Servings: 12

INGREDIENTS

2 cups almond flour

3 cage-free eggs

1 1/2 cups whole strawberries

1/4 cup sweetener*

1/4 cup coconut oil

2 teaspoons baking soda

1 teaspoon vanilla

1/2 teaspoon Celtic sea salt

INSTRUCTIONS

1. Preheat oven to 350 degrees F. Line 9 x 13 baking dish with parchment paper, or coat with coconut oil.

2. Add eggs to food processor or high-speed blender and process until light and thickened, about 1 minute. Remove stems from strawberries and roughly chop. Add to processor with sweetener, coconut oil and vanilla. Process until smooth.

3. Sift almond flour, baking soda and salt into medium mixing bowl. Pour in strawberry mixture and beat with hand mixer or whisk until well combined.

4. Pour batter into prepared baking pan and place in oven.

5. Bake 25 - 30 minutes, or until cake is golden brown on top and toothpick inserted into center comes out moist but clean.

6. Remove pan from oven and allow to cool 10 minutes.

7. Slice and serve warm. Or let cool completely and serve room temperature or warm.

NOTE: Line muffin pan with paper liners of light coat with coconut oil, fill 2/3 full with batter, and bake about 15 minutes for **Strawberry Cupcakes**.

stevia, raw honey or agave nectar

Orange Shortbread Cookies

Prep Time: 5 minutes

Cook Time: 20 minutes

Servings: 12

INGREDIENTS

1 1/2 cups almond flour

1/2 cup coconut flour

1/2 cup dried apricots

1/4 cup coconut oil (or melted cacao butter)

1 orange

1 lemon

1 teaspoon vanilla

1/4 teaspoon baking soda

1/4 teaspoon Celtic sea salt (plus extra)

INSTRUCTIONS

1. Preheat oven to 300 degrees F. Line sheet pan with parchment or baking mat.

2. Add apricots to food processor or bullet blender and process until coarsely ground. Or finely mince.

3. Add processed apricots to small mixing bowl. Zest *then* juice orange and lemon into bowl. Add oil or melted butter, and vanilla. Mix to combine.

4. Sift almond and coconut flour, baking soda and salt into medium mixing bowl. Pour wet ingredients into flour mixture and mix to form dough.

5. Use small scoop or tablespoon to drop portions of dough onto prepared sheet pan.

6. Place in oven and bake 20 minutes , or until lightly browned and firm.

7. Remove from oven and let cool at least 5 minutes.

8. Serve warm. Or let cool completely and serve room temperature.

Paleo Walnut Blast Cookies

Prep Time: 10 minutes

Cook Time: 15 minutes

Servings: 12

INGREDIENTS

3/4 cup almond flour

1/4 cup dried pitted dates

1/4 cup coconut oil

1/3 cup sweetener*

1 teaspoon vanilla

1 1/3 cup whole walnuts (3/4 cup chopped)

1 teaspoon baking powder

1/2 teaspoon baking soda

1/4 teaspoon Celtic sea salt

INSTRUCTIONS

1. Preheat oven to 350 degrees F. Line sheet pan with parchment or baking mat.
2. Add 1/2 cup whole or 1/3 cup chopped walnuts to food processor or high-speed blender. Process until finely ground.
3. Add ground walnuts to medium mixing bowl with almond flour, baking powder and soda, salt and vanilla. Whisk to lighten.
4. Add dates, coconut oil and sweetener to clean food processor or high-speed blender and process until smooth. Mix date mixture into flour mixture.

5. Chop whole walnuts (if using). Add chopped walnuts to bowl and mix until well combined.
6. Shape dough into 12 balls and place onto prepared baking sheet. Flattened slightly with hand or spatula.
7. Place in oven and bake 10 - 15 minutes, until golden browned along edges.
8. Remove from oven and let cool 5 minutes.
9. Serve immediately. Or transfer to wire rack to cool completely and serve room temperature.

raw honey, agave nectar or maple syrup

Chocolate Mint Cookies

Prep Time: 30 minutes

Cook Time: 15 minutes

Servings: 12

INGREDIENTS

Cocoa Lady Fingers

1/3 cup coconut flour

3 tablespoons arrowroot powder

4 cage-free eggs

1/4 cup sweetener*

2 tablespoons cocoa powder

1/2 teaspoon baking powder

1/2 teaspoon vanilla

Mint Chocolate Filling

4 oz organic dark chocolate

2 oz full-fat coconut milk

4 drops pure mint extract/oil

INSTRUCTIONS

1. Preheat oven to 400 degrees F. Line two sheet pans with parchment paper. Fit pastry bag with 1/2 inch round tip, or cut 1/4 inch corner off sturdy kitchen storage bag (like Ziploc®).

2. For *Cocoa Lady Fingers*, beat egg yolks, sweetener and vanilla until thick and pale.

3. In separate bowl, beat egg whites to stiff peaks with hand mixer or whisk, about 8 minutes.
4. Fold half of egg whites into egg yolk mixture. Then sift in coconut flour, cocoa, arrowroot powder and baking powder. Gently fold batter. Fold in remaining egg whites until mixture is uniform.
5. Scoop batter into pastry or storage bag. Place in tall round container and fold open end of bag over edge of container for easier prep.
6. Pipe 4 inch cookies onto prepared sheet pans about 2 inches apart.
7. Place in oven and bake for 8 minutes, until set and just golden.
8. Remove cookies from oven and transfer full parchment sheet onto wire rack to cool completely. Do not try to remove warm cookies from parchment.
9. Heat 1 inch of water in bottom of double boiler, or in bottom pan with metal or glass bowl on top.
10. For *Mint Chocolate Filling*, melt chocolate and coconut milk over double boiler until smooth. Remove from heat and stir in mint extract/oil.
11. Remove cooled *Cocoa Lady Fingers* from parchment. Dip bottom of cookie into chocolate mint mixture and press against bottom of second cookie to make sandwich. Repeat with remaining cookies.
12. Serve warm. Or let chocolate set for 10 minutes, in refrigerator if preferred, and serve chilled or room temperature.

*stevia, raw honey or agave nectar

Primal Pistachio Pinwheel Cookies

Prep Time: 10 minutes

Cook Time: 20 minutes

Servings: 12

INGREDIENTS

Dough

2 cups almond flour

2 tablespoon sweetener*

1 egg

1 teaspoon vanilla

1/2 teaspoon baking powder

1/4 teaspoon Celtic sea salt

Filling

1/2 cup shelled pistachios

2 tablespoons sweetener*

1/4 teaspoon ground ginger

1/2 teaspoon vanilla

INSTRUCTIONS

1. Preheat oven to 300 degrees F. Line sheet pan with parchment or baking mat. Prepare 2 additional sheets of parchment.

2. Place 1/4 cup pistachios in food processor or high-speed blender. Process until finely ground. Chop remaining pistachios, or crush with rolling pin between parchment sheets or in kitchen bag. Set aside.

3. For *Dough*, add flour, egg, sweetener, vanilla, baking powder and salt to medium mixing bowl. Blend with wooden spoon, then knead with hand to form thick dough.

4. Divide dough in half. Place half of dough in small mixing bowl. For *Filling*, add ground and chopped pistachios, sweetener, ginger and vanilla to small bowl. Mix until well combined.

5. Roll out each half of dough separately on parchment sheets. Roll into equal rectangles.

6. Place *Filling* rectangle on top of plain dough. Use parchment to help roll dough tightly along long edge into log.

7. Use sharp knife to cut log into 1/4 thick round slices. Place cookies on prepared sheet pan and bake about 10 minutes, until edges are golden brown.

8. Remove from oven and let cool about 5 minutes.

9. Serve warm. Or let cool completely and serve room temperature.

*raw honey, agave nectar or maple syrup

Paleo Angel Cake Delight

Prep Time: 15 minutes

Cook Time: 30 minutes

Servings: 12

INGREDIENTS

12 cage-free egg whites (room temperature)

1/2 cup sweetener*

3/4 cup arrowroot powder

1/4 cup coconut flour

1 1/2 teaspoons cream of tartar (optional)

1 teaspoon baking soda

1 1/2 teaspoons vanilla

1/4 teaspoon Celtic sea salt

INSTRUCTIONS

1. Preheat oven to 325 degrees F.
2. Sift arrowroot and coconut flour into small mixing bowl. Set aside.
3. In large mixing bowl, beat egg whites until they foam. Add baking soda, salt, vanilla and cream of tartar (optional). Beat egg whites well into soft peaks, about 5 minutes. Slowly drizzle in sweetener while beating to just under stiff peaks.
4. Gently fold four mixture into the egg whites with spatula.
5. Spoon batter into 6 - 8 ungreased mini tube or Bundt® pans. Use butter knife to cut through batter and make sure batter settles well into pans, then smooth tops.

6. Place pan on sheet pan and bake 20 - 25 minutes, or until top is golden brown and firm but springy.

7. Remove from oven and invert pans onto small raisers, like a butter knife or other small heatsafe object. This helps prevent the cakes from collapsing. Allow to cool completely

8. Serve room temperature.

raw honey or agave nectar

NOTE: Bake in Angel Food pan or tube pan for 1 hour for large **Angel Food Cake**.

Carrot Cake Cookie Bars

Prep Time: 10 minutes

Cook Time: 25 minutes

Servings: 12

INGREDIENTS

2 cups almond meal

2 cups shredded carrots (about 4 large carrots)

3 cage-free eggs

1/4 cup coconut oil

1/2 cup unsweetened applesauce

1/2 cup flaked coconut

1/4 cup sweetener*

2 teaspoons vanilla

2 teaspoons ground cinnamon

1 teaspoon ground nutmeg

1/2 teaspoon ground black pepper

1/2 teaspoon Celtic sea salt

INSTRUCTIONS

1. Preheat oven to 350 Degrees F. Line baking pan with parchment or coat lightly with coconut oil.

2. Grate carrots, or process in food processor or bullet blender until finely chopped. Add to medium bowl.

3. Add eggs, oil, applesauce and sweetener to food processor or bullet blender. Process until thickened and light, about 1 - 2 minutes.

4. Pour egg mixture into carrots. Sift in almond flour and salt. Add vanilla and spices. Mix well with a wooden spoon or hand mixer. Stir in coconut.

5. Press dough evenly into prepared baking pan and bake about 25 minutes, or until firm and golden brown.

6. Remove from oven and allow to cool about 10 minutes.

7. Slice into bars and serve warm. Or let cool completely and serve room temperature.

*stevia, raw honey, agave nectar or maple syrup

Lemon Spotted Muffins

Prep Time: 5 minutes

Cook Time: 20 minutes

Servings: 12

INGREDIENTS

6 cage-free eggs

1/2 cup coconut flour

1/4 cup coconut oil

1/4 cup sweetener*

1 teaspoon vanilla

1 teaspoon poppy seeds

1/2 teaspoon baking soda

Juice of 2 lemons

Zest of 2 lemons

INSTRUCTIONS

1. Preheat oven to 350 degrees F. Oil muffin pan or line with paper liners.
2. Zest, *then* juice 2 lemons. Add to large mixing bowl with eggs, coconut oil, sweetener and vanilla. Beat with hand mixer or whisk until well combined.
3. Sift coconut flour and baking soda into wet ingredients, and mix until smooth. Stir in poppy seeds.
4. Use ice cream scoop or tablespoon to pour batter into prepared muffin pan.

5. Place in oven and bake for about 20 minutes, or until golden around edges and toothpick inserted into middle comes out clean.

6. Remove from oven and let cool for 5 minutes.

7. Serve warm. Or allow to cool completely and serve room temperature.

raw honey or agave nectar

Paleo Coconut Macaroons

Prep Time: 10 minutes

Cook Time: 20 minutes

Servings: 12

INGREDIENTS

6 cage-free egg whites

3 cups flaked coconut

1/2 cup sweetener*

1 tablespoon coconut oil

1 teaspoon vanilla

1/4 teaspoon Celtic sea salt

INSTRUCTIONS

1. Preheat oven to 350 degrees F. Line a sheet pan with parchment paper or baking mat.

2. In large mixing bowl, beat room temperature egg whites with hand mixer to stiff peaks, about 7 - 8 minutes.

3. Beat in sweetener, vanilla and salt until combined. Fold in 1 cup of coconut at a time.

4. Use ice cream scoop or spoon to drop rounds of batter onto prepared sheet pan.

5. Bake for about 20 minutes, or until coconut is toasted and browned.

6. Allow to cool on pan for 10 minutes. Then remove from pan.

7. Serve warm. Or allow to cool completely and serve room temperature.

raw honey or agave nectar

Paleo Coconut Cake

Prep Time: 10 minutes

Cook Time: 25 minutes

Servings: 12

INGREDIENTS

Coconut Cake

6 cage-free eggs

3/4 cup coconut flour

1 cup flaked coconut

1 cup unsweetened applesauce

1/2 cup coconut oil

1/2 cup coconut milk

1/2 cup sweetener*

1/2 cup dried pitted dates

2 teaspoons vanilla

1 teaspoon baking soda

1 teaspoon baking powder

1/2 teaspoon Celtic sea salt

Coconut Frosting

1/3 cup coconut cream (from 1 can settled full-fat coconut milk)

2 - 4 tablespoons sweetener*

1/2 teaspoon vanilla

1/2 cup flaked coconut

INSTRUCTIONS

1. Preheat oven to 325°F. Line two or square baking pans with parchment or coat lightly with coconut oil.

2. Add dates, coconut milk, and half of eggs and oil to food processor or bullet blender. Process until dates a broken down, about 1 - 2 minutes.

3. Pour date mixture into medium bowl. Add applesauce, sweetener, vanilla, and remaining eggs and oil. Beat with hand mixer or whisk until well combined.

4. Sift coconut flour, salt, and baking soda and baking powder into wet ingredients. Blend until smooth. Stir in coconut.

5. Pour batter into prepared baking pans and bake for about 25 minutes, or until golden and toothpick inserted into center comes out clean.

6. Remove from oven and allow to cool. Place in refrigerator to speed cooling.

7. For *Coconut Frosting*, beat coconut cream in medium mixing bowl until slightly thickened. Add sweetener and vanilla, and continue to beat until full thickened and fluffy.

8. Frost cooled cakes and stack one on top of the other. Evenly sprinkle flaked coconut on top layer of frosted cake.

9. Slice and serve.

*stevia, raw honey, agave nectar or maple syrup

Everyday Recipes

Cave Style Breakfast Buns

Prep Time: 15 minutes

Cook Time: 20 minutes

Servings: 4

INGREDIENTS

Breakfast Bun

1 cup tapioca flour

1/4 - 1/3 cup coconut flour

1 cage-free egg

1/2 cup warm water

1/4 cup coconut oil

Bacon drippings

2 tablespoons applesauce

1 teaspoon apple cider vinegar

1/2 teaspoon baking soda

1/2 teaspoon ground black pepper

1/4 teaspoon Celtic sea salt

Filling

4 cage-free eggs

4 slices nitrate-free bacon

1/2 small bell pepper

1/2 small onion

1/4 teaspoon ground black pepper

1/4 teaspoon Celtic sea salt

INSTRUCTIONS

1. Preheat oven to 350 degrees F. Line sheet pan with parchment paper or coat with coconut oil. Heat medium skillet over medium-high heat. Add water to small pot and heat over medium heat.

2. For *Filling*, peel onion, stem, seed and vein pepper, and chop bacon. Add bacon to hot skillet and sauté until bacon is crisp and almost cooked through. Drain off drippings and set aside.

3. Dice onion and pepper and add to bacon. Sauté about 2 minutes, unto bacon is cooked through and veggies are softened. Add eggs and lightly scrambled, just 30 seconds - 1 minute. Remove from heat and set aside.

4. For *Breakfast Bun*, sift together tapioca flour, coconut flour, baking soda, salt and pepper in medium bowl.

5. Whisk egg, applesauce and vinegar in small bowl. Whisk in warm water, coconut oil and bacon drippings.

6. Add egg mixture to flour mixture and mix until well combined. Add 1 tablespoon coconut flour or water at a time if needed to form soft and slightly sticky dough.

7. Divide dough into 4 portions and flatten into round disks. Dust your hand or rolling pin with extra tapioca flour to prevent sticking.

8. Scoop loose egg *Filling* into center of each dough disk and pinch edges of dough together to create round, sealed ball.

9. Place filled buns sealed side down on sheet pan and pat down slightly.

10. Place in oven and bake 20 minutes, or until edges are golden brown and dough is cooked through.

11. Remove from oven and let cool about 5 minutes.

12. Serve warm.

Green Club Muffin

Prep Time: 10 minutes

Cook Time: 15 minutes

Servings: 12

INGREDIENTS

1 cup almond flour

2 cage-free eggs

1 avocado

4 slices nitrate-free bacon

1 tablespoon sweetener*

1 teaspoon apple cider vinegar

1 teaspoon baking powder

1/4 teaspoon ground white pepper (or black pepper)

INSTRUCTIONS

1. Preheat oven to 350 degrees F. Line muffin pan with paper liners or light coat with coconut oil. Heat medium pan over medium-high heat.

2. Finely chop bacon and add to hot pan. Sauté until crisp and cooked through, about 5 minutes. Set aside.

3. Beat eggs, sweetener and vinegar in medium mixing bowl with hand mixer or whisk until thick and slightly foamy.

4. Slice avocado in half. Scoop flesh of one half into egg mixture. Add bacon and drippings, almond flour, baking powder and black pepper and mix until combined.

5. Dice remaining avocado flesh and fold into batter.

6. Use ice cream scoop or tablespoon to scoop batter into prepared muffin pan.
7. Bake about 15 - 20 minutes, until edges are golden brown and tops are firm.
8. Remove from oven and let cool for 5 minutes.
9. Serve warm. Or cool completely and serve temperature.

NOTE: Bake in square oiled baking pan for 30 - 35 minutes for **Avocado Club Bread**.

stevia, raw honey or agave nectar

Primal Corn Muffins

Prep Time: 5 minutes

Cook Time: 15 minutes

Servings: 12

INGREDIENTS

1 cup almond flour

2 cage-free eggs

1/4 cup coconut oil

2 tablespoons unsweetened applesauce

1 teaspoon sweetener*

1 teaspoon organic apple cider vinegar

1 teaspoon baking powder

1/2 teaspoon ground turmeric (optional)

Pinch ground white pepper (optional)

INSTRUCTIONS

1. Preheat oven to 350 degrees F. Line muffin pan with paper liners or lightly coat with coconut oil.

2. Beat eggs in medium mixing bowl with hand mixer or whisk until thick and slightly frothy. Add oil, applesauce, sweetener, and vinegar and mix well.

3. Stir in almond meal, baking powder, and turmeric and white pepper (optional) until combined.

4. Use ice cream scoop or tablespoon to scoop batter into muffin pan, about 1/2 - 3/4 full.

5. Bake 15 - 18 minutes until edges are golden brown and the tops are firm.

6. Serve warm or room temperature.

NOTE: Bake in square oiled baking pan for 25 - 35 minutes for **"Corn" Bread**.

stevia, raw honey or agave nectar

Paleo English Muffins

Prep Time: 5 minutes

Cook Time: 15 minutes

Servings: 4

INGREDIENTS

1/3 cup coconut flour

4 cage-free eggs

1/4 cup almond milk (or low-fat coconut milk)

2 tablespoons coconut oil

1 tablespoon unsweetened applesauce

1/2 teaspoon baking soda

1 teaspoon organic apple cider vinegar

Pinch Celtic sea salt

INSTRUCTIONS

1. Preheat oven to 400 degrees F. Coat 4 mini-round cake pans or 4-inch diameter oven safe ramekins with coconut oil.
2. In small mixing bowl mix baking soda and apple cider vinegar together. Set aside and allow to froth.
3. In medium bowl, beat eggs with hand mixer or whisk until thick and frothy. Add flour, milk, applesauce and salt. Combine.
4. Add baking soda and vinegar mixture and blend well until smooth and free of clumps.
5. Pour batter into pans or ramekins and bake for 12 - 15 minutes, until slightly golden and center is firm to the touch.

6. Remove muffins from oven. Loosen from sides of pan or container with knife turn out.
7. Serve warm. Muffins will have traditional **English Crumpet** texture.

NOTE: For crusty, American style **English Muffins**, cut in half and toast in skillet coated with coconut oil. Press muffin down in pan with spatula and flip, browning on both sides.

stevia, raw honey or agave nectar

Coconut and Banana Pancake Supreme

Prep Time: 5 minutes

Cook Time: 15 minutes

Servings: 2

INGREDIENTS

Pancakes:

1 3/4 cups almond meal

1 teaspoon baking powder

2 cage-free eggs

3/4 cup coconut milk

1/4 cup flaked coconut

1/2 banana

1 teaspoon vanilla

1/4 teaspoon Celtic sea salt

Coconut oil (for cooking)

Topping:

1/2 banana

Agave nectar (optional)

INSTRUCTIONS

1. Heat a large skillet over medium-high heat and lightly coat with coconut oil.

2. Mash 1/2 banana in medium bowl with fork. Whisk in eggs, then coconut milk and vanilla.

3. Add almond flour, salt and baking powder. Whisk until smooth. Fold in coconut flakes.

4. Use ladle or dry measure cup to pour 1/4 cup of batter onto hot oiled skillet. Fit 2 or 3 pancakes comfortably, so they do not touch as they spread.

5. Cook until sides of pancakes are firm and batter bubbles up a bit. About 3 to 4 minutes.

6. Carefully flip pancakes with spatula and cook for additional minute, or until cooked through. Repeat with remaining batter. Re-oil pan if necessary. Pancakes will be slightly delicate, so flip and plate with care.

7. Slice 1/2 banana. Top with banana slices and agave nectar. Serve warm.

Ultimate Bacon & Fruit Scramble

Prep Time: 10 minutes

Cook Time: 15 minutes

Servings: 2

INGREDIENTS

6 cage-free eggs

4 slices nitrate-free bacon

2 dried figs

1 sweet apple

1 bell pepper

1 small sweet onion

1/2 teaspoon ground black pepper

1/2 teaspoon paprika

1/2 teaspoon Celtic sea salt

1/2 teaspoon cinnamon (optional)

INSTRUCTIONS

1. Bring small pot to boil with lightly salted water. Heat medium skillet over medium-high heat.

2. Dice bacon and add to hot skillet. Brown bacon for about 3 minutes, stirring occasionally with wooden spatula.

3. Add figs to boiling water for 5 minutes.

4. Peel and core apple. Stem and seed pepper. Peel onion. Dice apple, pepper and onion and add to skillet. Sauté another 2 minutes, until veggies caramelize and bacon crisps.

5. Remove figs from boiling water and dice. Add to skillet, plus spices. Sauté another minute.

6. Crack eggs directly into skillet and scramble gently with wooden spatula.

7. Cook eggs to desired firmness and serve hot.

Paleolithic Egg Bread

Prep Time: 15 minutes

Cook Time: 20 minutes

Servings: 4

INGREDIENTS

3 cups almond flour

6 cage-free egg yolks (room temperature)

3 cage-free eggs (room temperature)

1/2 cup coconut oil

1/4 cup sweetener*

1 tablespoon apple cider vinegar

1 teaspoon baking soda

1/2 teaspoon Celtic sea salt

1 cage-free egg

INSTRUCTIONS

1. Preheat oven to 350 degrees F. Coat muffin pan with coconut oil or line with paper liners. Cover cutting board with parchment.

2. Add eggs and yolks to large mixing bowl. Beat with hand mixer or whisk until light and frothy. Beat in coconut oil, sweetener, vinegar, baking soda and salt. Sift in 2 1/2 cups almond flower while mixing to form sticky dough.

3. Dust parchment covered cutting board with remaining almond flour. Turn dough out onto parchment and knead for about 5 minutes.

4. Transfer dough to prepared muffin pan. Beat remaining egg in small mixing bowl and brush over bread.

5. Place in oven and bake 15 - 20 minutes, until browned and cooked through.

6. Remove from oven and let cool for 5 minutes.

7. Serve warm. Or allow to cool completely and serve room temperature.

stevia, raw honey or agave nectar

NOTE: Bake in oiled loaf pan for 40 minutes for **Egg Bread Loaf**, or form ropes and braid dough together then bake on prepared sheet pan for 30 minutes for **Classic Egg Bread**.

Green Crush Smoothie

Prep Time: 5 minutes

Servings: 2

INGREDIENTS

2 cups spinach

2 whole kale leaves (1 cup chopped)

1 banana

1 green apple

1/2 cup green grapes

1 cup water (or fresh nut milk)

INSTRUCTIONS

1. Remove stems and ribs from kale. Core apple and dice. Peel banana.
2. Add water, banana and grapes to full sized blender. Process until solids are broken down.
3. Add greens and pulse on low for 30 seconds to break down. Then process on high for 1 minute, until smooth.
4. Pour into serving glasses and serve immediately.
5. Or chill in refrigerator for 20 minutes, blend for a few seconds to incorporate separated liquid, then pour into serving glasses and serve chilled.

Red Berry Blast Smoothie

Prep Time: 5 minutes

Servings: 1

INGREDIENTS

1 cup strawberries

1/2 cup red raspberries

1/4 cup pitted cherries

1/4 cup cherry tomatoes

1/2 - 1 cup water (or fresh nut milk)

Juice of 1 beet (optional)

INSTRUCTIONS

1. Remove leaves from strawberries and chop. Add to full sized blender with raspberries, cherries, tomatoes and beet juice (optional).

2. Add 1/2 cup water and pulse on low for 30 seconds to break down. Add more water if necessary. Then process on high for 30 seconds to 1 minute, until smooth.

3. Pour into serving glasses and serve immediately.

4. Or chill in refrigerator for 20 minutes, blend for a few seconds to incorporate separated liquid, then pour into serving glasses and serve chilled.

Strawberry Banana Swirl Shake

Prep Time: 5 minutes*

Cook Time: 0 minutes

Servings: 1

INGREDIENTS

1 banana

1 cup strawberries

1/2 - 1 cup water

Meat of 1/2 fresh coconut (or 1/2 cup unsweetened flaked or shredded coconut)

INSTRUCTIONS

1. *Soak flaked coconut in water for at least 4 hours.
2. Add fresh or soaked flaked coconut and water to high-speed blender. Process on high until smooth, about 1 minute.
3. Strain coconut mixture through nut milk bag or a few layers of cheese cloth. Squeeze out all excess liquid. Reserve coconut milk. Dry excess coconut, process until finely ground, and use as coconut flour.
4. Remove leaves from strawberries and chop. Peel banana.
5. Add coconut milk to blender with fruit and process on high until smooth.
6. Pour into serving glass and serve immediately.
7. Or chill in refrigerator for 20 minutes, blend for a few seconds to incorporate separated liquid, then pour into serving glass and serve chilled.

Cashew Butter Banana Sandwich

Prep Time: 10 minutes

Cook Time: 20 minutes

Servings: 4

INGREDIENTS

Sandwich Bread

1 cup tapioca flour/starch

1/4 - 1/3 cup coconut flour

1 cage-free egg

1/2 cup warm water

1/4 cup coconut oil

1/4 cup applesauce

1 tablespoon sweetener*

1 teaspoon apple cider vinegar

1/2 teaspoon baking soda

1/2 teaspoon cinnamon

1/2 teaspoon Celtic sea salt

Filling

1/2 cup cashews (raw or roasted)

2 tablespoons coconut oil

1 tablespoon sweetener*

1/4 teaspoon cinnamon

1 banana

INSTRUCTIONS

1. Preheat oven to 350 degrees F. Line sheet pan with parchment paper or coat with coconut oil.

2. In medium bowl, sift together tapioca flour, 1/4 cup coconut flour, baking soda and salt. Stir in warm water and oil.

3. Whisk egg in small bowl. Add applesauce, vinegar and cinnamon. Add egg mixture to flour mixture and mix until well combined. Add 1 tablespoon coconut flour or water at a time if needed to form soft and slightly sticky dough.

4. Divide dough into 4 portions and roll into round or oval balls. Dust your hand with extra tapioca flour to prevent sticking.

5. Place rolls on sheet pan and pat down slightly. Bake 20 minutes, or until edges are golden brown and the tops are firm. Remove from oven and allow to cool.

6. While *Sandwich Bread* is baking, add cashews, coconut oil, sweetener and cinnamon to food processor or bullet blender and process until smooth. Add 1/2 tablespoon of coconut oil at a time if necessary to reach preferred consistency. Or use jarred cashew butter.

7. Slice bananas. Slice cooled *Sandwich Bread* in half and spread on cashew butter. Layer banana slices on bread.

8. Serve immediately. Or wrap in plastic wrap or parchment and store in lidded container.

*stevia, raw honey or agave nectar

Strawberry Swirl Sandwich

Prep Time: 10 minutes

Cook Time: 20 minutes

Servings: 4

INGREDIENTS

Sandwich Bread

1 cup tapioca flour/starch

1/4 - 1/3 cup coconut flour

1 cage-free egg

1/2 cup warm water

1/4 cup coconut oil

1/4 cup applesauce

1 tablespoon sweetener*

1 teaspoon apple cider vinegar

1/2 teaspoon cinnamon

1/4 teaspoon ground ginger

1/2 teaspoon baking soda

1/2 teaspoon Celtic sea salt

Filling

1/2 cup almonds (raw or roasted)

2 tablespoons coconut oil

1 tablespoon sweetener*

1/4 teaspoon cinnamon

1/4 teaspoon ground ginger

5 - 6 medium strawberries

INSTRUCTIONS

1. Preheat oven to 350 degrees F. Line sheet pan with parchment paper or coat with coconut oil.

2. In medium bowl, sift together tapioca flour, 1/4 cup coconut flour, baking soda and salt. Stir in warm water and oil.

3. Whisk egg in small bowl. Add applesauce, vinegar, cinnamon and ginger. Add egg mixture to flour mixture and mix until well combined. Add 1 tablespoon coconut flour or water at a time if needed to form soft and slightly sticky dough.

4. Divide dough into 4 portions and roll into round or oval balls. Dust your hand with extra tapioca flour to prevent sticking.

5. Place rolls on sheet pan and pat down slightly. Bake 20 minutes, or until edges are golden brown and the tops are firm. Remove from oven and allow to cool.

6. While *Sandwich Bread* is baking, add almonds, coconut oil, sweetener, cinnamon and ginger to food processor or bullet blender and process until smooth. Add 1/2 tablespoon of coconut oil at a time if necessary to reach preferred consistency. Or use jarred almond butter.

7. Slice strawberries. Slice cooled *Sandwich Bread* in half and spread on almond butter. Layer strawberry slices on bread.

8. Serve immediately. Or wrap in plastic wrap or parchment and store in lidded container.

*stevia, raw honey or agave nectar

Primal Beef Bun

Prep Time: 15 minutes

Cook Time: 30 minutes

Servings: 4

INGREDIENTS

Bun

1 cup tapioca flour/starch

1/4 - 1/3 cup coconut flour

1 cage-free egg

1/2 cup warm water

1/2 cup coconut oil

1 teaspoon apple cider vinegar

1/2 teaspoon baking soda

1 teaspoon Celtic sea salt

Filling

8 oz ground beef

1/2 small onion

1 garlic clove

1 teaspoon ground cumin

1/2 teaspoon chili powder

1/4 teaspoon cayenne

1/2 teaspoon ground black pepper

1/2 teaspoon Celtic Sea salt

INSTRUCTIONS

1. Preheat oven to 350 degrees F. Line sheet pan with parchment paper or coat with coconut oil. Heat medium skillet over medium-high heat.

2. For *Filling*, grind or mince onion and add to skillet with beef, salt and spices. Sauté until cooked through and browned, about 8 - 10 minutes. Remove from heat and set aside.

3. In medium bowl, sift together tapioca flour, 1/4 cup coconut flour, baking soda and salt. Stir in warm water and oil.

4. Whisk egg and vinegar in small bowl. Add egg mixture to flour mixture and mix until well combined. Add 1 tablespoon coconut flour or water at a time if needed to form soft and slightly sticky dough.

5. Divide dough into 4 portions and flatten into round disks. Dust your hand or rolling pin with extra tapioca flour to prevent sticking.

6. Scoop beef filling into center of dough disks and pinch edged of dough together to create round, sealed ball.

7. Place buns sealed side down on sheet pan and pat down slightly. Bake 20 minutes, or until edges are golden brown and dough is cooked through.

8. Serve immediately. Or store in lidded container.

Mighty Onion Crumpets

Prep Time: 5 minutes

Cook Time: 15 minutes

Servings: 4

INGREDIENTS

1/3 cup coconut flour

4 cage-free eggs

1/4 cup nut milk

2 tablespoons coconut oil

1 tablespoon unsweetened applesauce

1/2 teaspoon baking soda

1 teaspoon organic apple cider vinegar

1 teaspoon onion powder

1/4 teaspoon Celtic sea salt

1 teaspoon dehydrated onion flakes (optional)

INSTRUCTIONS

1. Preheat oven to 400 degrees F. Coat 4 mini-round cake pans or 4-inch diameter ramekins with coconut oil.

2. In small mixing bowl, mix baking soda and apple cider vinegar. Set aside and allow to froth.

3. In medium bowl, beat eggs with hand mixer or whisk until thick and lightened. Add flour, nut milk, applesauce, onion powder and salt. Mix to combine.

4. Add baking soda and vinegar mixture to medium bowl. Blend well until smooth.

5. Pour batter into prepared pans or ramekins and sprinjle on dehydrated onion flakes (optional). Bake for 12 - 15 minutes, until slightly golden and center is firm to the touch.

6. Remove muffins from oven. Loosen from sides of pans or ramekins with knife, then turn out.

7. Serve warm. Or let cool complete and serve room temperature.

Jalapeño Lime Comfort Pretzel

Prep Time: 15 minutes

Cook Time: 20 minutes

Servings: 4

INGREDIENTS

1 cup coconut flour

1/2 cup tapioca flour

1/2 cup coconut oil

1/2 cup water

1 cage-free egg

Juice of 1/2 lime

Zest if 1/2 lime

1 fresh jalapeño (or 2 oz pickled jalapeño)

2 tablespoons apple cider vinegar

1/2 teaspoon baking soda

1/2 teaspoon baking powder

1/2 teaspoon Celtic sea salt

Cilantro Lime Almond Cheese

1 cup soaked, skinless almonds*

3/4 cup water

1 tablespoons coconut oil

Juice of 1/2 lime

1 clove garlic

1/2 teaspoon Celtic sea salt

Pinch ground black pepper

Small bunch cilantro

1 1/2 cups water (for soaking)

INSTRUCTIONS

1. *Soak almonds in 1 1/2 cups water overnight. Drain and remove skins.
2. Preheat oven to 350 degrees F. Heat medium pot over medium-high heat. Line sheet pan with parchment or baking mat.
3. Add coconut oil, water, vinegar and salt to pot. Bring to a boil and remove from heat.
4. Whisk in tapioca flour. Stir with wooden spoon or soft spatula until mixture gels and comes together.
5. Stir in baking soda and baking powder. Mix for 1 minute. Mixture will foam and expand. Let mixture sit and cool about 5 minutes.
6. Remove stem, seed and veins from jalapeño and mince. Zest lime into pot, then add juice and jalapeño. Mix to incorporate.
7. Sift in coconut flour. Mix partially, then beat in egg. Blend until combined. Excess coconut flour may sit in bottom of bowl.
8. Turn out dough onto cutting board dusted with any excess coconut flour from mixture. Knead dough for 2 minutes.
9. Cut dough into 4 equal portions. Roll out pieces into ropes and twist to form classic pretzel twist. Pinch together any crumbled dough.
10. Arrange pretzels on lined sheet pan. Brush with coconut oil or full-fat coconut milk for glossy finish.
11. Place sheet pan in oven and bake about 25 minutes, until cooked through and golden.

12. For *Lime Almond Cheese*, peel garlic and add to food processor or high-speed blender with soaked almonds, coconut oil, lime juice, cilantro, salt and pepper. Process until smooth. Add water as necessary to reach desired consistency. You may process, let it rest, then process again to reach desired consistency.

13. Transfer *Cilantro Lime Almond Cheese* to serving dish.

14. Remove pretzels from oven and serve warm with *Cilantro Lime Almond Cheese*.

Cave Style Thai Curry

Prep Time: 20 minutes

Servings: 2

INGREDIENTS

1 tomato

1 carrot

1/2 red pepper

1/2 lemon

1/2 mango

2 cups cauliflower florets

1/2 small onion

1 teaspoon Celtic sea salt

Coconut Curry Sauce

1/2 cup fresh coconut

1/2 lemon

1 lemongrass stem

1 inch piece fresh ginger

1 garlic clove

1 tablespoon fresh curry leaves

Medium bunch fresh parsley

1/2 teaspoon red pepper flakes

1 teaspoon Celtic sea salt

Water

INSTRUCTIONS

1. Seed and chop bell pepper. Seed tomato if preferred, then chop. Dice carrot. Add to medium mixing bowl. Add juice of 1/2 lemon and 1/2 teaspoon salt. Mix and set aside.

2. For *Coconut Curry Sauce*, peel ginger and garlic. Remove coconut flesh from shell and chop. Remove half of parsley from stem. Add to food processor or high-speed blender with lemongrass, lemon juice, curry leaves, salt and red pepper. Process until smooth and creamy, about 1 - 2 minutes. Add enough water to reach desired consistency.

3. Add *Coconut Curry Sauce* to mixing bowl with veggies. Toss to coat and refrigerate at least 10 minutes.

4. Peel onion. Add cauliflower and onion to food processor with shredding attachment and process to "rice." Or mince cauliflower and onion. Add to medium mixing bowl with 1/2 teaspoon salt and mix to combine.

5. Cut mango in half around pit, peel and dice. Chop remaining parsley.

6. Plate "rice" mixture and top with *Coconut Curry Sauce* . Sprinkle mango and parsley over curry. Serve immediately.

Simple Cashew Curry

Prep Time: 10 minutes*

Servings: 2

INGREDIENTS

2 cups cauliflower florets

1 banana

1 teaspoon Celtic sea salt

1/2 cup raw cashews

Water

Cashew Curry Sauce

1/2 cup raw cashews

1/2 red bell pepper

1 small leek

2 teaspoon coconut aminos (or tamari)

Juice of 1/2 lemon

2 teaspoons curry powder

1 teaspoon ground turmeric

1/4 teaspoon cayenne pepper

1/4 teaspoon Celtic sea salt

Water

INSTRUCTIONS

1. *Soak 1/2 cup cashews in enough water to cover over night in refrigerator. Drain and rinse.

2. For *Cashew Curry Sauce*, add cashews to food processor or high-speed blender and process until finely ground.

3. Seed and chop bell pepper. Chop leek. Add to ground cashews with coconut aminos, lemon juice, salt and spices. Process until smooth and creamy, about 1 - 2 minutes. Add enough water to reach desired consistency.

4. Add cauliflower to food processor with shredding attachment and process to "rice." Or mince cauliflower and add to medium mixing bowl with 1/2 teaspoon salt and mix to combine.

5. Peel banana and dice.

6. Plate "rice" mixture and top with diced banana and soaked cashews. Top with *Cashew Curry Sauce*. Serve immediately.

Easy Pesto Caprese Salad

Prep Time: 5 minutes

Servings: 2

INGREDIENTS

1 large yellow tomato

1 large red tomato

Small bunch fresh basil

Celtic sea salt, to taste

Crack or ground black pepper, to taste

Basil Pesto

2 cups basil leaves (packed)

1/4 cup raw pine nuts

1/2 - 1/3 cup raw oil (coconut, walnut, almond, sesame, etc.)

2 garlic cloves

1/2 lemon (or 1 tablespoon raw apple cider vinegar)

1/4 teaspoon Celtic sea salt

INSTRUCTIONS

1. For *Basil Pesto*, peel garlic and add to food processor or high-speed blender with squeeze of 1/2 lemon. Process until finely chopped. Add pine nuts, basil, oil and salt and process until finely ground, about 1 minute.

2. Slice tomatoes and plate in alternating colors. Sprinkle with salt and pepper. Chiffon basil leaves.

3. Spread *Basil Pesto* over tomato slices and top with fresh basil. Serve immediately.

Ultimate Primal Pad Thai

Prep Time: 10 minutes

Servings: 1

INGREDIENTS

1 medium zucchini

1 large carrot

1 green onion (scallion)

1/2 cup purple cabbage (shredded)

1/2 cup cauliflower florets

1/2 cup mung bean or radish sprouts (optional)

Large bunch cilantro

1/3 cup raw almonds

Raw Pad Thai Sauce

2 tablespoons raw tahini (or 3 tablespoons raw sesame seeds)

2 tablespoons raw nut butter (or 1/4 cup raw nuts)

1 tablespoon lime juice (or lemon juice)

2 tablespoons coconut aminos (or tamari or raw apple cider vinegar)

1 tablespoon sweetener*

1 small garlic clove

1/4 inch piece fresh ginger

INGREDIENTS

1. Use spiralizer, mandolin, vegetable peeler or grater to thinly
   slice zucchini and carrot. Add to medium bowl. Shred cabbage

and slice green onion. Chop cauliflower and cilantro. Add to bowl with sprouts (optional).

2. Add almonds to food processor or high-speed blender and pulse to coarsely grind. Set aside.

3. For *Raw Pad Thai Sauce*, peel ginger and garlic. Add to food processor or high-speed blender with tahini and nut butter, or sesame seeds and nuts, lime juice, coconut aminos and sweetener. Process until smooth and creamy, about 1 - 2 minutes.

4. Add to veggies and toss to coat. Transfer to serving dish and sprinkle on ground almonds. Serve immediately.

*stevia, raw honey or dried dates

Zesty Clam Dish

Prep Time: 5 minutes*

Servings: 1

INGREDIENTS

12 large little neck clams

3/4 lemon

Raw Cocktail Sauce

1 large tomato

Juice of 1/4 lemon

2 tablespoons raw sesame seeds(or 1 tablespoon raw tahini)

1 tablespoon fresh ground horseradish

Pinch Celtic sea salt

Pinch cracked black pepper

INSTRUCTIONS

1. Have fishmonger shuck clams. *Or carefully shuck clams yourself.
2. Arrange clams around serving dish.
3. Add sesame seeds to food processor or high-speed blender and process until smooth, if using.
4. Or seed tomato and add to processor or blender with tahini, lemon juice, horseradish, salt and pepper. Process until smooth and transfer to small serving bowl.
5. Serving clams with *Raw Cocktail Sauce* immediately.

Southwestern Chili

Prep Time: 10 minutes*

Servings: 2

INGREDIENTS

5 - 6 plum tomatoes

1/2 teaspoon dried cumin

1/4 teaspoon chili powder

1/4 teaspoon onion powder

1/4 teaspoon garlic powder

1 teaspoon fresh oregano leaves (or 1/4 teaspoon dried oregano)

1/2 teaspoon ground black pepper

1/4 teaspoon cayenne pepper or red pepper flakes (optional)

1 teaspoon Celtic sea salt

1 teaspoon chia seed (or flax seed)

1/2 cup raw cashews

Water

INSTRUCTIONS

1. *Soak raw cashews in enough water to cover overnight in refrigerator. Drain and rinse. Set aside.

2. Grind chia or flax in food processor or high-speed blender. Set aside.

3. Juice tomatoes. Or add to food processor or high-speed blender and process. Add enough water to reach desired consistency, if necessary. Then strain.

4. Add tomato juice, ground chia or flax, 1/2 of soaked cashews, salt, pepper and spices to blender. Process until smooth, about 1 - 2 minutes.

5. Stir in remaining soaked cashews.

6. Pour into serving bowls and serve immediately.

Paleo Broccoli Creamy Soup

Prep Time: 10 minutes*

Servings: 2

INGREDIENTS

1 1/2 - 2 cups broccoli florets

1 red bell pepper

1 garlic clove

1/4 cup raw oil (coconut, walnut, almond, sesame, etc.)

1 cup nutritional yeast

1 tablespoon coconut aminos (or tamari)

1 tablespoon onion powder

1/2 teaspoon Celtic sea salt

1/4 teaspoon ground white pepper (or ground black pepper)

2 cups raw cashews

Water

INSTRUCTIONS

1. * Soak raw cashews in enough water to cover at least 2 hours, or overnight in refrigerator. Drain and rinse. Set aside.
2. Chop broccoli florets into pieces and set aside.
3. Seed and vein bell pepper. Peel garlic. Add to food processor or high-speed blender with soaked cashews, nutritional yeast, coconut aminos, salt, pepper and enough water to process until smooth, about 2 - 3 minutes.
4. Pour into serving bowl and top with broccoli. Serve immediately.

Primal Raspberry Fusion Salad

Prep Time: 10 minutes

Servings: 1

INGREDIENTS

Salad

2 cups soft lettuce leaves (looseleaf or butterhead varieties)

1/2 cup watercress

2 tablespoons raw almonds (slivered or sliced)

1/4 cup fresh raspberries

Raspberry Vinaigrette

1/4 cup raspberries (fresh or frozen)

2 tablespoons lemon juice (or raw apple cider vinegar)

2 tablespoons raw walnuts (or raw walnut oil, coconut oil, almond oil, etc.)

1 teaspoon sweetener* (optional)

Water

INSTRUCTIONS

1. For *Salad*, rinse, dry and plate lettuce and watercress. Sprinkle almonds and fresh raspberries over greens.
2. For *Raspberry Vinaigrette*, add raspberries, lemon juice, walnuts or oil, and sweetener (optional) to food processor or high-speed blender and process until smooth, about 1 minute. Add enough water to reach desired consistency.

3. Drizzle *Raspberry Vinaigrette* over salad and serve immediately.

*stevia, raw honey or dried dates

Cave People Guacamole

Prep Time: 5 minutes

Cook Time: 5 minutes

Servings: 4

INGREDIENTS

2 avocados

1 shallot

1 small tomato

1 bunch cilantro

Half lime

2 teaspoons paprika

1/2 teaspoon ground cumin

1/2 teaspoon ground black pepper

1/2 teaspoon Celtic sea salt

INSTRUCTIONS

1. Peel and finely dice shallot. Dice tomato and cilantro. Add to small mixing bowl.
2. Slice avocados in half, pit, and scoop flesh into bowl. Add 1 teaspoon paprika, 1/2 teaspoon cumin, 1/2 teaspoon black pepper and 1/2 teaspoon salt.
3. Mash avocado and mix ingredients well with fork. Transfer to serving dish and squeeze on juice of half a lime. Sprinkle with remaining teaspoon of paprika.
4. Serve immediately. Or refrigerate 30 minutes, and serve chilled.

Rugged Coconut Shrimp

Prep Time: 10 minutes

Cook Time: 15 minutes

Servings: 4

INGREDIENTS

3 cage-free egg whites

1 lb large shrimp

1 cup flaked coconut

1/2 teaspoon garlic powder

1/2 teaspoon ground white pepper (or ground black pepper)

1 teaspoon Celtic sea salt

Coconut oil (for cooking)

Mango Salsa

1 ripe mango

1/2 small white onion

1 small jalapeño

Juice of half lime

INSTRUCTIONS

1. Preheat oven to 425 degrees F. Line sheet pan with parchment paper. Or place oven-safe wire rack over sheet pan.
2. Add coconut to shallow dish.
3. Beat egg whites with salt, pepper and garlic powder in a large mixing bowl with hand mixer or whisk until light and fluffy.

4. Peel and devein shrimp. Leave tails on. Add shrimp to egg whites to coat.

5. Let excess egg white drain from shrimp, then add to coconut flakes. Toss to coat. Return shrimp to egg whites, then coconut flakes again. Press shrimp into coconut and coat well.

6. Place the shrimp on prepared sheet pan. Brush lightly with liquid coconut oil.

7. Place in oven and bake for 5 - 7 minutes. Then turn shrimp over, brush with coconut oil, and bake another 5 - 7 minutes, until coconut is golden brown and shrimp are bright pink.

8. For *Mango Salsa*, slice mango around pit. Peel and dice flesh. Peel and dice onion. Mince jalapeño, discarding seeds and stem. Add to small serving dish juice of half a lime. Mix to combine.

9. Remove shrimp from oven and allow to cool for a few minutes.

10. Serve warm with *Mango Salsa*.

Toasty Almond Cream Cakes

Prep Time: 15 minutes*

Cook Time: 20 minutes

Servings: 12

INGREDIENTS

Cake

1 cup almond flour

4 cage-free egg whites

1/3 cup coconut oil

1/4 cup almond milk

1/4 cup sweetener*

1 teaspoon baking powder

1/4 cup slice almonds

Almond Cream

2 cups skinless almonds

1/4 cup sweetener

1 teaspoon vanilla

Water

INSTRUCTIONS

1. *Soak almonds overnight in water. Drain and rinse.
2. Preheat the oven to 350 degrees F. Heat medium pan over medium heat. Lightly coat muffin pan with coconut oil, or line with paper liners

3. Add almond flour to hot dry pan and toast about 5 minutes, stirring frequently. Do not burn. Remove from heat and set aside.

4. Beat egg whites to soft peaks with hand mixer or whisk in medium bowl. Then beat in oil, milk and 1/4 cup sweetener. Sift in toasted almond flour and baking powder. Mix until just combined.

5. Use ice cream scoop or spoon to scoop batter into muffin pan. Each cup should be only 1/2 full.

6. Bake about 15 minutes, or until center is set but springy.

7. Remove pan from oven and remove cakes from pan. Let cool for about 15 minutes.

8. While cakes cool, blend soaked almonds, 1/4 cup sweetener, 1 teaspoon vanilla and water as needed in food processor or blender to make smooth *Almond Cream*.

9. Wipe out pan with paper towel and return dry pan to medium heat. Toast slice almonds about 5 minutes, until aromatic and golden. Do not burn. Remove from heat and set aside.

10. When cakes are cooled, slice in half to create top and bottom layer. Scoop cream onto bottom half, and top with top half of cake. Scoop another dollop of cream over top half and sprinkle on slice toasted almonds.

11. Serve room temperature.

NOTE: For large **Toasted Almond Cream Cake** , bake batter in 2 round cake pans for 35 - 40 minutes.

* raw honey, agave nectar or maple syrup

Classic Pineapple Upside Down Cake

Prep Time: 15 minutes

Cook Time: 30 minutes

Servings: 12

INGREDIENTS

2 cups almond flour

8 - 12 slices organic canned pineapple in juice

8 - 12 pitted cherries

1/4 cup sweetener*

3 cage-free eggs

1/4 cup coconut oil

1/2 cup organic pineapple juice (reserved from can)

2 teaspoons baking soda

2 teaspoons vanilla

1/2 teaspoon Celtic sea salt

INSTRUCTIONS

1. Preheat oven to 350 degrees F. Line 9x13 baking dish with parchment paper, or coat with coconut oil.
2. Arrange pineapple slices and cherries on bottom of baking dish. Place in oven while you prepare the batter.
3. Beat egg whites to stiff peaks with hand mixer or whisk in medium mixing bowl. About 7 - 10 minutes.
4. In large mixing bowl, mix yolks, olive oil, sweetener, pineapple juice and vanilla.

5. Sift almond flour, baking soda and salt into yolk mixture. Beat until well combined.
6. Fold egg whites into batter until evenly combined.
7. Remove hot baking pan from oven, and spread light batter over pineapple and cherries. Smooth top with spatula.
8. Bake for 25 - 30 minutes, or until cake golden brown and firm but springy in the center. A toothpick inserted into the center should come out clean.
9. Remove pan from oven and allow to cool for 15 minutes. Turn cake out onto serving dish and remove parchment. Or scrape any stuck fruit from the pan and place back on cake.
10. Allow to cool another 15 minutes before serving. Serve room temperature or warm.

NOTE: For **Pineapple Upside Dow Cupcakes** , add a pineapple slice and cherry to muffin pan lined with paper liners or coated with coconut oil, then fill cups 2/3 full with batter and bake about 20 minutes.

stevia, raw honey or agave nectar

Banana Bread Pudding Delight

Prep Time: 10 minutes

Cook Time: 30 minutes

Servings: 12

INGREDIENTS

Banana Bread

1 cup of almond flour

2 cage-free eggs

2 overripe bananas

1/4 cup sweetener*

2 tablespoons coconut oil

1 tablespoon baking powder

1 tablespoon cinnamon

1 teaspoon nutmeg

1 teaspoon vanilla

1/2 teaspoon of Celtic sea salt

Banana Custard

13 oz (1 can) full-fat coconut milk

6 cage-free egg yolks

1 overripe banana

1/4 cup sweetener*

1/4 cup raisins

1/2 cup dried pitted dates

2 tablespoons tapioca starch/flour

2 teaspoons vanilla

1 teaspoon cinnamon

Pinch Celtic sea salt

INSTRUCTIONS

1. Preheat oven to 350 degrees F. Line muffin pan with paper liners or coat with coconut oil.

2. In medium mixing bowl, beat 2 eggs, 2 bananas, 2 tablespoons oil and 1/4 cup sweetener with hand mixer or whisk.

3. In separate mixing bowl, add 1 cup almond flour, 1 tablespoon baking powder,1 tablespoon cinnamon, 1 teaspoon nutmeg, 1 teaspoon vanilla and 1/2 teaspoon salt.

4. Pour banana mixture into flour mixture and mix well.

5. Pour batter into muffin pan and bake for about 15 minutes, or until golden brown, risen and firm.

6. While muffins cook, add coconut milk, egg yolks, banana, sweetener, vanilla, cinnamon and salt to medium bowl and blend briefly with hand mixer or whisk.

7. Pour into medium pot and heat over medium heat. Chop dates and add to pot with raisins.

8. Stir in tapioca flour. Stir as *Banana Custard* thickens, about 5 minutes. Remove from heat.

9. Remove muffins from oven and turn out onto cutting board.

10. Increase oven to 375 degrees F. Lightly coat square or rectangular baking dish with coconut oil.

11. Carefully remove paper liners and roughly chop muffins. Add muffin chunks to baking dish. Pour banana custard over chopped muffins.

12. Place dish in oven and bake for 15 minutes.

13. Remove and allow to cool for 15 minutes before serving.

14. Serve warm or room temperature.

*stevia, raw honey or agave nectar

Simply Sweet Potato Blondie Refresher

Prep Time: 15 minutes

Cook Time: 30 minutes

Servings: 12

INGREDIENTS

2/3 cups coconut flour

2 tablespoons arrowroot powder

1 large sweet potato

4 cage-free eggs

3/4 cup sweetener*

1/4 cup full-fat coconut milk

1/4 cup cacao butter

1/2 teaspoon baking powder

2 tablespoons vanilla

Pinch Celtic sea salt

Pinch ground white pepper (or black pepper)

INSTRUCTIONS

1. Preheat oven to 350 degrees F. Grease an 9 x 13 inch pan or "all-corner" specialty brownie pan with coconut oil. Bring medium pot of lightly salted water to boil.

2. Peel and dice sweet potato. Add to boiling water for 5 - 10 minutes, until soft.

3. Beat eggs in medium mixing bowl with hand mixer or whisk. Add sweetener, coconut milk, vanilla and pepper until combined.

4. Sift in flour, arrowroot powder, baking powder and salt, and mix until combined.

5. Drain sweet potatoes and add to small mixing bowl with cacao butter. Beat or mash until cacao butter is well melted. Add sweet potato mixture to egg mixture.

6. Scrape batter into baking pan and smooth top with spatula.

7. Bake for 25 - 30 minutes, until center is firm and top is golden brown. Toothpick inserted into center will come out moist but mostly clean.

8. Allow to cool about 10 minutes. Slice and serve warm or room temperature.

*stevia, raw honey or agave nectar

Coconut Cream Comfort Pie

Prep Time: 20 minutes*

Cook Time: 20 minutes

Servings: 8

INGREDIENTS

Crust

1/2 cup soft nuts**

1 cup almond flour

2 teaspoons sweetener***

1/4 - 1/2 cup coconut oil

Filling

26 oz (2 cans) full-fat coconut milk

2 cage-free eggs

1/2 cup arrowroot powder

1/4 cup sweetener*

1 tablespoon vanilla

1 cup flaked coconut

Pinch Celtic sea salt

INSTRUCTIONS

1. Preheat oven to 350 degrees F. Lightly coast pie plate with coconut oil.

2. Grind nuts into coarse meal with food processor or bullet blender. Add to small bowl with almond flour, 2 tablespoons

sweetener and enough coconut oil to bring together soft but crumbly dough.

3. Press dough into pie plate and bake about 10 - 15 minutes, until crust becomes golden.

4. Remove crust from oven and allow to cool. Turn off oven.

5. Add coconut milk, eggs, arrowroot powder, sweetener, vanilla and salt to medium pot. Heat pot over medium heat and bring to a boil. Stir constantly as mixture thickens.

6. Stir in 1/2 cup shredded coconut. Then pour the filling over the crust.

7. *Refrigerate pie until filling is set, about 4 hours.

8. Heat medium pan over medium heat. Add 1/2 cup flaked coconut and toast about 5 minutes. Stir frequently to prevent burning.

9. Sprinkle toasted coconut over pie and serve chilled.

NOTE: Line springform pan with parchment and bake crust, then fill with coconut cream filling for another version of **Coconut Cream Pie**.

*coconut flakes, pecans, walnuts, cashews or brazil nuts
**stevia, raw honey or agave nectar

Paleo Strawberry Bread

Prep Time: 10 minutes

Cook Time: 10 minutes

Servings: 12 - 16

INGREDIENTS

1 cup coconut flour

3/4 cup cashew flour (or almond flour)

1/4 cup ground chia seed (or flax meal)

1/2 cup coconut oil

2 cage-free eggs

1/4 cup coconut crème

1/4 cup sweetener*

1/4 cup unsweetened apple sauce

1 teaspoons baking powder

1 tablespoon ground cinnamon

1 teaspoon ground ginger

1 teaspoon ground white pepper (or black pepper)

1 teaspoon Celtic sea salt

2 cups fresh sliced strawberries

1/2 cup chopped walnuts (optional)

INSTRUCTIONS

1. Preheat oven to 350 degrees F. Line muffin pan with paper liners or coat with coconut oil.

2. In large bowl, whisk eggs with hand mixer or whisk until frothy and light. Add coconut oil, sweetener and applesauce.

Blend until combined. Slice strawberries, and fold in with walnuts (optional).

3. In medium bowl, blend flours, chia meal, baking powder, salt and spices. Stir flour blend into strawberry mixture until well combined.

4. Use ice cream scoop or tablespoon to scoop equal portions of batter into muffin pans, 1/2 - 3/4 full. Line or oil more muffin pans if excess batter remains.

5. Bake for 15 minutes, or until golden brown and firm but springy to the touch.

6. Cool enough to handle. Serve warm or room temperature.

NOTE: Bake in square oiled baking pan for 25 - 35 minutes or two oiled loaf pans for 35 - 45 minutes for **Strawberry Loaves**.

*stevia, raw honey or agave nectar

Primal Apple Cider Bread

Prep Time: 10 minutes

Cook Time: 20 minutes

Servings: 24

INGREDIENTS

2 cups coconut flour

1 cup almond flour

12 ounces organic hard cider

2 cage-free eggs

1/2 cup unsweetened applesauce

1 tart apple

2 tablespoons baking powder

1 teaspoon ground nutmeg

1 teaspoon ground black pepper

1 teaspoon Celtic sea salt

INSTRUCTIONS

1. Preheat oven to 375 degrees F. Line 2 muffin pans with paper liners or coat with coconut oil.

2. Peel, core and grate or dice apple, and place in large bowl. Pour hard apple cider over apples, plus nutmeg and black pepper.

3. In medium bowl, whisk eggs with hand mixer or whisk until frothy and light. Add applesauce and blend until combined. Add egg mixture to cider and apples.

4. Slowly sift and stir flours, baking powder and salt into wet ingredients.

5. Use ice cream scoop or tablespoon to scoop equal portions of batter into muffin pans, 1/2 - 3/4 full.

6. Bake for 15 - 20 minutes, or until golden brown and firm but springy to the touch.

7. Cool enough to handle. Serve warm or room temperature.

NOTE: Bake in square oiled baking pan for 35 - 45 minutes or two oiled loaf pans for 45 - 55 minutes for **Primal Apple Cider Loaves**.

*stevia, raw honey or agave nectar

Mandarin Pumpkin Coconut Bread

Prep Time: 5 minutes

Cook Time: 25 minutes

Servings: 12

INGREDIENTS

1 3/4 cups coconut flour

2 cage-free eggs

1/4 cup coconut oil

1/2 cup coconut milk

1/2 unsweetened applesauce

1/4 cup sweetener*

15 oz (1 can) pumpkin puree

2 teaspoons baking soda

1 tablespoon ground cinnamon

1 teaspoon ground nutmeg

1 teaspoon Celtic sea salt

1/2 cup flaked coconut

1/4 cup pumpkin seeds

Water

INSTRUCTIONS

1. Preheat oven to 350 degrees F. Coat square baking pan with coconut oil.

2. Process eggs, coconut oil, coconut milk, applesauce and sweetener in food processor or blender until thick and

lightened. Pour into medium mixing bowl. Mix in pumpkin puree and spices.

3. Mix in flour, baking soda, flaked coconut and pumpkin seeds. Stir until combined.

4. Pour batter into oiled baking pan. Bake 20 - 25 minutes, or until firm but springy in center.

5. Serve warm or room temperature.

NOTE: Bake in lined or oiled muffin pan for 15 - 20 minutes for **Pumpkin Coconut Muffins**.

*stevia, raw honey or agave nectar

Garlic Goodness Rolls

Prep Time: 10 minutes

Cook Time: 20 minutes

Servings: 6

INGREDIENTS

1 cup tapioca flour/starch

1/4 - 1/3 cup coconut flour

1 cage-free egg

1/2 cup warm water

1/4 cup coconut oil

1/4 cup unsweetened applesauce

1/2 teaspoon baking soda

1 teaspoon apple cider vinegar

2 garlic cloves

Small bunch fresh basil

1 teaspoon dried parsley

1 teaspoon rosemary

Small pinch fresh marjoram (optional)

1/2 teaspoon ground black pepper

1 teaspoon Celtic sea salt

INSTRUCTIONS

1. Preheat oven to 350 degrees F. Line sheet pan with parchment paper or coat with coconut oil.

2. Whisk egg in small bowl. Peel and mince garlic, plus rosemary, fresh basil and marjoram (optional). Whisk applesauce, vinegar, garlic and fresh herbs into egg.

3. In medium bowl, blend tapioca flour, 1/4 cup coconut flour, baking soda, salt and dried spices. Stir in warm water and oil. Add egg mixture and mix until well combined.

4. If necessary, add coconut flour or water 1 tablespoon at a time to form soft and slightly sticky dough.

5. Use ice cream scoop or large spoon to scoop out 6 portions of dough and roll into round or oblong balls. Dust hands with extra tapioca flour to prevent sticking.

6. Place rolls on sheet pan and pat down slightly. Bake 20 minutes, or until edges are golden brown and tops are firm. Serve warm or room temperature.

NOTE: For **Garlic 'N Herb Italian Bread**, roll dough into single log and bake at 325 degrees F for 30 - 35 minutes, or until outside is toasted and center is cooked through.

Savory Tomato Rolls

Prep Time: 10 minutes

Cook Time: 20 minutes

Servings: 6

INGREDIENTS

1 cup tapioca flour/starch

1/4 - 1/3 cup coconut flour

1 cage-free egg

1/2 cup warm organic tomato sauce

1/4 cup coconut oil

1/4 cup fresh tomato puree (or minced tomato flesh, no skin)

1/2 teaspoon baking soda

1 teaspoon apple cider vinegar

1 teaspoon dried basil

1 teaspoon dried oregano

1/2 teaspoon ground black pepper

1/2 teaspoon Celtic sea salt

INSTRUCTIONS

1. Preheat oven to 350 degrees F. Line sheet pan with parchment paper or coat with coconut oil.

2. Process fresh skinned tomato flesh in food processor or bullet blender. Or mince. Whisk egg in small bowl. Whisk in fresh tomato and vinegar.

3. In medium bowl, blend tapioca flour, 1/4 cup coconut flour, baking soda, salt and spices. Stir in warm tomato sauce and oil. Add egg mixture and mix until well combined.

4. If necessary, add coconut flour or water 1 tablespoon at a time to form soft and slightly sticky dough.

5. Use ice cream scoop or large spoon to scoop out 6 portions of dough and roll into round or oblong balls. Dust hands with extra tapioca flour to prevent sticking.

6. Place rolls on sheet pan and pat down slightly. Bake 20 minutes, or until edges are golden brown and tops are firm. Serve warm or room temperature.

NOTE: For **Savory Tomato French Bread**, roll dough into single long log and bake at 325 degrees F for 30 - 35 minutes, or until outside is toasted and center is cooked through.

Blueberry Blast Blondies

Prep Time: 10 minutes

Cook Time: 30 minutes

Servings: 12

INGREDIENTS

4 cage-free eggs

3/4 cup coconut flour

2 tablespoons arrowroot powder (or tapioca flour)

1 cup (1/2 pint) fresh blueberries

1/2 cup sweetener*

1/4 cup full-fat coconut milk

1/2 teaspoon baking powder

2 teaspoons vanilla

1 teaspoon food-grade lavender buds (ground)

1/2 teaspoon Celtic sea salt

INSTRUCTIONS

1. Preheat oven to 350 degrees F. Coat rectangular baking pan or "all-corner" specialty brownie pan with coconut oil.

2. Add blueberries to food processor or bullet blender with coconut milk and process until smooth. Set aside.

3. Beat eggs in medium mixing bowl with hand mixer or whisk. Add blueberry purée, sweetener, vanilla and lavender. Mix to combine.

4. Sift coconut flour, arrowroot or tapioca, baking powder and salt into blueberry mixture. Beat until well combined.

5. Scrape batter into prepared baking pan and smooth top with spatula.

6. Bake for 25 - 30 minutes, until center is firm and top is golden brown. Toothpick inserted into center will come out moist but mostly clean.

7. Remove from oven and allow to cool about 10 minutes.

8. Slice and serve warm. Or allow to cool completely and serve room temperature.

stevia, raw honey or agave nectar